Cognitive Aids to Support
Health Professionals

Health and Patients Set

coordinated by
Bruno Salgues

Volume 5

Cognitive Aids to Support Health Professionals

Thierry Morineau

Foreword by Dr. Morgan Jaffrelot

ISTE

WILEY

First published 2024 in Great Britain and the United States by ISTE Ltd and John Wiley & Sons, Inc.

ISTE Ltd
27-37 St George's Road
London SW19 4EU
UK

www.iste.co.uk

John Wiley & Sons, Inc.
111 River Street
Hoboken, NJ 07030
USA

www.wiley.com

Library of Congress Control Number: 2024937865

British Library Cataloguing-in-Publication Data
A CIP record for this book is available from the British Library
ISBN 978-1-78630-954-9

Contents

Foreword

We might have assumed that beyond the surgical checklist, the notion of cognitive assistance would lead us far from our caregiving concerns. However, Thierry Morineau, a (deeply) engaged professor of ergonomics, both in the academic curriculum of health science students and in the daily routines of healthcare providers, elucidates in this volume the significance of cognitive aids within the healthcare domain. This book will provide insights for healthcare professionals in their daily practice. Furthermore, it will enlighten managers, be they administrative or caregiving. Ultimately, it is poised to assist health science educators in raising awareness among healthcare providers about the intricate interplay between individuals and their surroundings throughout both initial training and ongoing education programs. Through the diverse perspectives offered in this book, and depending on their stance towards care contexts, readers can discover "psychological instruments" (to take one of the concepts presented) to contemplate the multifaceted aspects of cognitive aids.

Healthcare professional

The healthcare provider will be capable of assessing both the vulnerability and the resilience of their reasoning in a given situation. Implicit within the text, we comprehend the fragility of an individual's reasoning at times and the imperative to assist them in maintaining accurate perception of the situation and in decision-making. Presently, there is scant emphasis in healthcare provider curricula on explaining cognitive vulnerability. Implicitly, the culture of "zero tolerance" for errors still prevails. Teaching clinical reasoning, including its vulnerabilities and biases, is now an essential requirement (Pelaccia 2016a; Audétat et al. 2017).

Confronted with this acknowledged vulnerability, the concept of "cognitive aid" must carve out a role within the action process. Analogous to a pilot facing a critical situation, such as an engine fire, who necessarily engages in automatic actions followed by written checks before relying on a to-do list, healthcare providers should be able to reference a notebook in critical scenarios without being suspected of incompetence. Regrettably, ingrained habits prove challenging to alter, and the management of risk and error in the healthcare domain is still nascent. Encouragingly, this cultural shift can occur organically within teams, on the ground, fostering awareness of underlying issues, devising novel workflows and integrating cognitive aids into their practice. Consequently, the team can serve as a cognitive aid unto itself for healthcare providers (Kahneman et al. 2021).

Manager

In hospital management, a critical misunderstanding revolves around the role ascribed to service protocols and procedural documents. Their functions, as well as those of data collection sheets, often harbor ambiguity and consequently are poorly grasped by healthcare providers. Regrettably, these documents are frequently viewed solely through the lens of activity tracking, overlooking their potential to assist professionals in avoiding errors during cognitive overload. "Protocols remain tucked away in binders while monitoring sheets serve merely to trace healthcare providers". Such critical disparities between what is prescribed and what is actually implemented may stem from protocols that are challenging to understand and ill-suited to the real-life contexts of healthcare providers' work. Therefore, there is a need to design user-friendly documents that actively support action. To achieve this goal, Thierry Morineau proposes a co-design approach involving future users, aiming to initiate a gradual process of appropriation.

Teacher

Contemporary trends in pedagogy underscore the significance of developing contextualized teaching methodologies to facilitate the transfer of learning (Vanpee et al. 2009). In this regard, teacher training cannot overlook an understanding of ergonomics. It involves drawing insights from this discipline to analyze and characterize professional scenarios based on work analysis methods. Prioritizing the identification of *key contextual elements* within which actions are performed will enable the prioritization of those elements that need to be taught (didactic translation). This, in turn, requires implementing a pedagogical transposition to organize teaching, learning and assessment activities effectively (Parent and Jouquan 2013).

The cognitive analysis of work, as presented in the book through the TMTA (Turing Machine Task Analysis) method, enables the identification of key information involved in triggering knowledge schemas or heuristics.

This approach is particularly relevant for educators engaged in health simulation development, providing valuable insights for enhancing scenario design. Indeed, the analysis of activity (whether prior to or provoked during debriefing) allows us to transcend the apparent realism and similarity of a simulated (reconstructed) situation, aiding in a deeper understanding of its authenticity from the learners' perspective. Understanding the challenges involved in solving a healthcare problem may lead to identifying vulnerabilities that could be mitigated through cognitive assistance. Considering the role of external cognition in reasoning does not mean losing sight of internal cognition; rather, it involves integrating it into the broader cognitive system that emerges from the interaction between individuals and their environment. This facilitates the development of a dynamic appropriation of procedural, conditional and declarative knowledge.

Cognitive aid as a Turing machine

However, how can we conceptualize a cognitive aid that provides the necessary and sufficient information to progress through a protocol and meet the support needs of users in context? By depicting a cognitive aid like a Turing machine, the second part of the book offers concrete proposals by characterizing:

– a working document like a Turing machine tape that is read by an agent to find information supporting their activity;

– a network of mental states to navigate through to ensure adherence to a protocol or work procedure.

Cognitive aids range from very simple to highly sophisticated information systems. The Turing machine model serves to unify all of these systems, enabling them to be understood as genuine cognitive aids in a given situation.

Keywords...

Another point of entry into the book could be through keywords. Indeed, aside from certain professions (such as occupational therapists, psychomotor therapists, physiotherapists) where ergonomics (especially physical) is taught, ergonomics (especially cognitive) remains a discipline that is rarely emphasized in health science studies. Yet, today, concepts and issues such as *human factors*, *contextualized teaching and learning*, *mental load*, the need for *cognitive gateways*, the *relevance* of cognitive aids, the *degree of coupling between the healthcare provider and the situation*, *modes of analytical and intuitive thinking*, *work analysis*, gaps between *prescribed tasks* and *real activity*, the awareness of internal cognition, as well as *cognition inscribed within the working environment*, are integral components of a health professional's daily environment.

This book as a gateway

So, how to use this book. For some, it serves as an introduction to ergonomics, while for others, it functions as a compendium of experiments and studies aimed at illustrating methods for designing, testing and using cognitive aids.

As an educator, I can only express gratitude to Thierry Morineau for his significant contribution to the healthcare provider community. Through his exploration, he forges a link between ergonomics and healthcare. Consequently, this book prompts numerous questions that emerge upon reading: How can students be trained in the use of cognitive aids? What role should these aids play in health sciences curricula? Answers to these questions unfold through the pages of this indispensable resource, serving as both a cornerstone in the field and a catalyst for creativity.

Morgan JAFFRELOT
Emergency Physician
Associate Professor in the Department of Anesthesiology and Intensive Care
Université Laval, Quebec
Teaching Assistant in the Master 2 Program in Health Sciences Pedagogy
CFRPS, University of Strasbourg

Acknowledgments

This book could not have come to fruition without the wealth of exchanges and collaborations from which I have so fully benefited with healthcare providers, health educators, healthcare executives and managers, particularly within the Ponchaillou University Hospital in Rennes, the B3S Simulation Center at the Centre Hospitalier de Bretagne Sud in Lorient, the Centre Hospitalier Bretagne Atlantique, the Saint-Avé Public Mental Health Institution, the Morbihan Medical-Psychological Emergency Unit, the Normandy Medical-Psychological Emergency Unit, the Morbihan Emergency Care Teaching Center and also within the Vannes Institute for the Training of Health Professionals, where I was graciously accommodated for two years within its team.

This book was also able to draw on the trust of partners such as the National Research Agency, the National Network of Maisons des Sciences de l'Homme, the Maison des Sciences de l'Homme of Brittany, the Brittany region, the Biotech Santé Bretagne, the company Excense, the National Center for Space Studies (CNES), AirZeroG and, of course, the Bretagne Sud University and the team at the LP3C (Psychology Laboratory: Cognition, Behaviour and Communication).

Finally, my gratitude extends to Morgan Jaffrelot, who graciously shared his insightful perspective on healthcare professionals and provided valuable guidance towards certain lines of reflection that proved to be fruitful during the writing of this book. For this English edition, it was a genuine pleasure to benefit from the expertise and positive demeanor of Ms. Nivetha Velupur, the translator.

Introduction

> "Working is a favor when it helps us think about what we are doing."
>
> Mossi Proverb, West African People

Patient safety is closely linked to the quality of the working conditions of healthcare professionals. A challenging environment for healthcare professionals is a source of errors, as it induces discomfort, stress and fatigue. Workplace hardship is defined in the French Labor Code as encompassing three factors:

– physical constraints: handling loads, awkward postures, vibrations, etc.;

– a harsh physical environment: toxic chemical agents, noise, ambient temperature, etc.;

– the pace of work: night work in successive and alternating shifts, repetitive work, etc.

The working conditions of many healthcare professionals often "tick" these three boxes, making this sector particularly demanding. To improve these working conditions, *physical ergonomics*[1] (analyzing gestures and postures, environmental factors such as acoustics, lighting, temperature, etc.) provides concepts, methods and recommendations that can lead to design or redesign proposals for a given workstation. Using physical ergonomics means both providing solutions to

1 Ergonomics (or *human factors*) is defined as "the scientific discipline that seeks to understand the fundamental interactions between humans and the other components of a system, and the profession that applies theoretical principles, data, and methods to optimize the well-being of individuals and the overall performance of systems" (IEA n.d.).

healthcare professionals and reducing the likelihood of adverse events affecting the health of caregivers and patients.

However, discomfort, stress and fatigue – the primary stressors generated by unsuitable working conditions – may also be linked to another aspect of the job. This other aspect pertains to the informational environment in which healthcare professionals are immersed. Information from patients, colleagues or an increasing number of information systems, coupled with a substantial amount of knowledge required to comprehend each care situation, often leads to an excessively high mental workload. The influx of information from transmitters and receivers (patients, colleagues, alarms, phone calls, etc.) interrupts tasks or time-sharing, disrupting trains of thought. This over-solicitation of mental activity poses risks of forgetfulness or confusion, potentially resulting in errors. Here, cognitive ergonomics, a branch of ergonomics, can offer concepts, methods and ultimately solutions to facilitate information management, reduce psychological discomfort, mental fatigue, stress and error frequency. Moreover, it has been established that musculoskeletal disorders can be caused not only by improper gestures, postures and work rhythms but also by cognitive and/or psychological overexertion (ANACT 2008; Zelano 2014). In other words, the issue of physical strain intersects with that of mental strain.

Concretely, *one way to improve the informational working environment is to make cognitive aids available to caregivers*. Cognitive aids are intended to relieve the mental workload[2], reduce the risks associated with task interruptions or multitasking contexts, and ensure care reliability with regard to good practices. Also, if a cognitive aid is not yet available "off the shelf", it is possible to design one from scratch. Health professionals and managers of medical facilities obviously did not wait for ergonomists to design their cognitive aids. However, it is necessary to emphasize that the implementation of a cognitive aid is not an insignificant intervention. It is a journey fraught with pitfalls that, in some cases, can lead to devices that, despite the laudable intentions of their designers, do not achieve their objectives or even constitute an additional constraint leading to explicit or implicit rejection by users. To achieve an effective means of improving the cognitive conditions of work, a cognitive aid must undergo in-depth reflection regarding its purposes and the consequences on the work situation. The pitfalls that cognitive aid designers face are potentially multifold. They can arise from doubts or even negative prejudices within teams regarding the impact of such a device on their working

2 Workload encompasses both physical and mental (or cognitive) loads. It refers to the resources mobilized to meet the demands imposed by the execution of a task (Leplat 1977).

conditions. Paradoxically, designers may also struggle with their own biases regarding the ease of developing an aid and the assurance of achieving a positive impact on working conditions.

We will have the opportunity to elaborate on the barriers that have been observed in the field during the integration of a new cognitive aid. However, we can already mention the bureaucratic aspect of a cognitive aid embedding itself in the format of a new form in daily activities. On a workstation already burdened with multiple constraints, adding what would be an additional constraint is inherently very risky, and in this regard, we can fully understand the apprehensions of future users regarding a new work document, whether it is in paper or digital format.

Other blocking points can arise from the unwise enthusiasm that designers invest in their cognitive aid projects. Many cognitive aids used in the field of health or in other domains, where safety and complexity issues to be managed are equally crucial, are manifested through a simple sheet of paper on which instructions are to be followed or information is to be verified. Taking the example of the checklist, which represents the "primary" cognitive aid in the workplace, it essentially involves ticking a series of checkboxes on a piece of paper. For a cognitive aid designer, this implies that merely writing on a sheet placed on the edge of a table, based on their personal representation of work, is sufficient to create a cognitive aid.

Another false hope, more sophisticated in nature, involves the mere transfer, without adaptation, of cognitive aids used in other domains, such as aeronautics, directly to the realm of healthcare, with the expectation of yielding effective devices. While, as we will explore, endeavors in risk management and cognitive aid design originating from aeronautics have indeed facilitated, and continue to facilitate, substantial advancements in the healthcare sector, these endeavors do not provide comprehensive solutions. Healthcare professionals undeniably encounter specific work constraints distinct from those of airplane pilots. Therefore, it is imperative to acknowledge and address these constraints accordingly.

Confronted with these potential pitfalls, intentionally exaggerated here to underscore them, as well as numerous other pitfalls worthy of recognition, the reader must be cautioned that cognitive ergonomics[3] does not offer ready-made solutions for designing cognitive aids. In this book, we will explore ergonomic recommendations, albeit primarily limited to providing general advice on

3 Cognition can be defined as the collection of information processing operations conducted by a living organism or an artificial agent, including perception, reasoning, memorization, planning, etc. Cognition is distinguished from affective and conative processes (will and motivation).

information presentation within a working document. The contributions of ergonomics are primarily elsewhere.

Conceptually, cognitive ergonomics, rooted in cognitive psychology, demonstrates how cognitive aids naturally integrate into human information processing strategies on a daily basis, functioning as psychological instruments.

Through its theoretical assumptions, cognitive ergonomics posits that a workstation or service fundamentally constitutes a system with a certain dynamic equilibrium point. Consequently, the introduction of a new cognitive aid involves a transient imbalance, ultimately leading to the establishment of a new equilibrium point that may not necessarily be more satisfactory than the previous one.

Finally, a crucial contribution of cognitive ergonomics lies in the methodological realm. While general recommendations often have limited applicability, analysis of the work practices of prospective users of cognitive aids is an essential method to ensure that the device meets the needs of the field and does not become an additional constraint imposed upon the work system.

The aim of this book is to illustrate the various contributions of cognitive ergonomics for both designers and users of cognitive aids. The initial phase of this inquiry centers on the fundamental objectives of cognitive aids (Part 1). From this foundation, the specific functions of individual cognitive aids are delineated (Chapter 1). It becomes apparent that cognitive aids serve as conduits between an individual's internal cognition and the external cognition embedded within the environment (Chapter 2). While knowledge often resides initially within the minds of healthcare providers, the implementation of cognitive aids facilitates the transfer of this knowledge to the external environment, thus engendering distributed cognition. Moreover, the introduction of cognitive aids frequently involves a shift in information processing strategies among users, transitioning from intuition-based reasoning to the analytical thinking facilitated by cognitive aids (Chapter 3). Nonetheless, it is also demonstrated that a move towards increased intuition, facilitated by certain aids, can be both feasible and beneficial (Chapter 4). Furthermore, cognitive aids serve as frameworks for providing directives and work procedures, thereby integrating into communication methods for instructing personnel navigating the complexities of real-world constraints (Chapter 5).

Lastly, the reader will discover methodological elements for designing a cognitive aid as a comprehensive information system, capable of providing fundamentally relevant information (Part 2). This objective will involve modeling cognitive aids as Turing machines. Consequently, a cognitive aid can be conceptualized as both a strip of tape used by an agent to store information (Chapter 6) and/or as a network of mental states of the agent using this tape (Chapter 7). Each perspective will bring forth its array of methods and techniques for work analysis, reasonably enabling us to aspire to devices that genuinely enhance the working conditions of healthcare professionals and, consequently, the modalities of patient care.

PART 1

Cognitive Aid as a Gateway

Introduction to Part 1

Health cognitive aids represent one of the significant outcomes of the development of risk management policies in healthcare facilities. It is noteworthy that risk management policies offer an original perspective on adverse events that may arise within a healthcare service, a viewpoint that is not to be taken for granted. No longer is it solely about interpreting the sudden deterioration of a patient's condition as merely reflecting the natural progression of their illness, the limitations of medical intervention in restoring health or attributing it to errors made by individual caregivers due to their lack of expertise. Instead, risk management encourages viewing adverse events as indicators, among other factors, of the vulnerability inherent in the overall work system in which these events occur. This approach involves adopting a systemic outlook on healthcare delivery and necessitates sufficient detachment from the emotions evoked by a patient's death, as well as from the conventional inclination to assign blame according to principles of individual legal responsibility.

Opting for a systemic interpretation of an adverse event involves understanding this event as *a consequence of the context in which patient care was administered.* This context, which forms the daily working conditions for medical and paramedical caregivers, comprises multiple components, complicating the analysis. Moreover, within the system, information circulates between individuals, within the same individual throughout tasks, and during interactions with materials and diverse physical environments. Consequently, the operational dynamics of a healthcare delivery system result from numerous interactions among these components, generating information that requires processing.

When considering this systemic perspective, coupled with the notion that the fundamental benchmark for assessing the effective functioning of a system is the individuals comprising it, we arrive at an approach referred to as the "human factors" approach. Once this viewpoint is embraced, attention can be directed towards the challenge of designing a cognitive aid within the work system. The design objective will be to ensure the long-term reliability of certain information flows, extending beyond specific events. This may involve tasks such as verifying the operational status of medical equipment, facilitating access to care protocols or enhancing communication quality within a team. Designing a device with consideration for how operators process information within a work system constitutes *cognitive engineering.*

Throughout the first part of the book, we will delve into a pivotal aspect of the design process: the question of what purpose a cognitive aid serves, its objective. For instance, a cognitive aid may aim to store information in hardware memory, deemed more resilient than healthcare providers' short-term memory, especially under time constraints. However, a potential pitfall arises when viewing cognitive aids solely as compensatory tools for caregivers lacking in information processing skills or rationality. Through this lens, cognitive aids risk being perceived merely as vehicles for delivering more information, fostering logical reasoning and promoting standardization in judgments and decisions. There is even the danger of them being seen as replacements for caregivers, assuming some of their responsibilities. Caregivers, susceptible to cognitive biases, may overly rely on vague intuitions, hunches or ingrained habits, deviating dangerously from protocols and directives issued by the hierarchy through official documents.

By regarding cognitive aids as mere instruments among others, distinguished by their ability to serve as gateways that facilitate the transfer of cognitive resources from various internal or external sources to the individual within the work system, constructive advancements can be made in proposing cognitive aids that are tailored to work contexts. Positioned as an instrument, cognitive aids act as intermediaries between caregivers and their working environment. In this initial section of the book, the examination of various definitions of cognitive aids within the framework of risk management, along with a thorough exploration of the gateway concept, will enable us to explain the fundamental purposes of cognitive aids.

1

Defining a Cognitive Aid

In defining cognitive aids, we will begin with the notion that they are devices designed to bolster mental activity in order to prevent failure. This definition is rooted in the historical adoption of the concept of cognitive aids within the hospital domain. Subsequently, we will explore a definition that regards cognitive aids as instruments among others, subject to ergonomic criteria. The integration of these two definitions will culminate in the proposal of a novel third definition, conceiving cognitive aids as pathways for cognition.

1.1. Cognitive aid as a support device for mental activity

Defining a cognitive aid as a support device for mental activities offers a clear advantage: it is a definition that is both simple and intuitive, being the first to come to mind. *A cognitive aid serves to facilitate, ensure reliability and enhance the security of task execution by addressing perception, reasoning, memory, decision-making and action planning.* Cognitive aids can support one or more stages of information processing to prevent omissions and failures.

To examine the integration of a work aid within mental activity more precisely, cognition can be conceptualized as a chain of information processing with its stages. The double-scale decision model proposed by Rasmussen (1986) illustrates such a processing chain (Figure 1.1).

This processing chain consists of several major phases, comprising mental states and mental operations:

– phase 1: perception of the situation for identification of the state of the world (activation of the perceptual system, observation of the detected data, identification);

– phase 2: development of a mental model for decision-making, task definition (interpretation of this state of the world and evaluation of alternatives for decision-making);

– phase 3: decision and execution of a task (definition of a task, formulation of the task in terms of procedure, execution of actions);

– in addition to these three phases, it is possible to include cross-sectional short-term or long-term memorization operations.

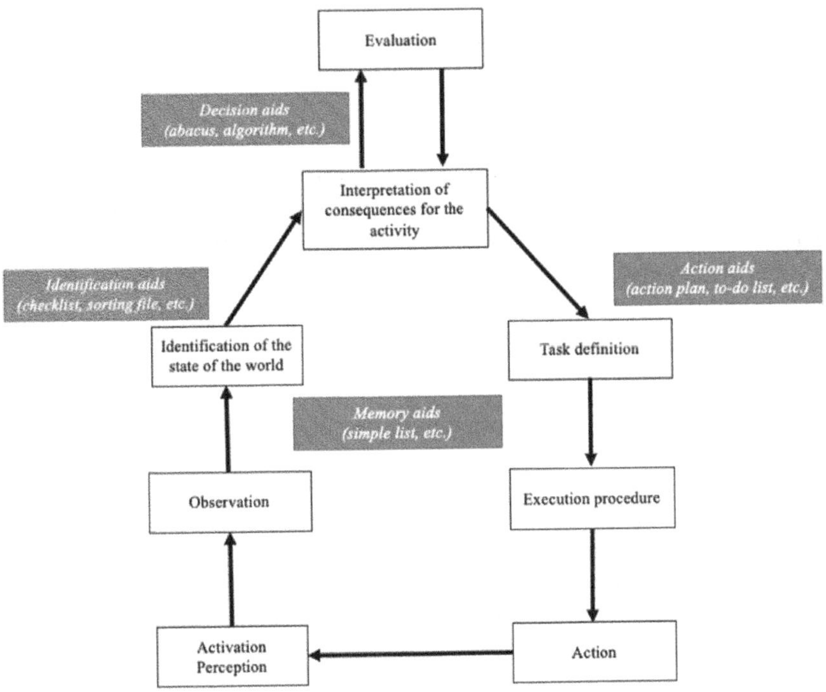

Figure 1.1. *Simplified double-scale decision model (adapted from Rasmussen (1986)) with the types of cognitive aids supporting the stages of information processing*

The processing phases are interconnected in the logic of the "perception–action" cycle, meaning that the execution of actions by an individual (phase 3) alters the state of the world and thus their perception of the situation, leading to the analysis of new information (phase 1). Based on each of these information processing phases, three types of cognitive aids can be distinguished. These aids contribute to achieving the outcome expected from each phase of information processing.

– *Identification aids:* these are the devices that facilitate the identification of the state of the situation and the assessment of its components. The *checklist* is a typical example.

– *Decision aids:* by proposing alternatives or linking the state of the world with decisions to be made, these aids provide support in defining tasks to be carried out. Examples include a chart showing the evolution of sizes and weights in children or, in a more sophisticated manner, software using artificial intelligence.

– *Action aids:* a list of actions to be carried out (*to-do list*), a working procedure describing the steps to be followed during the execution of a task guides the execution of actions.

– *Memory aids:* recording information on a paper or digital document brings with it a function of storing information that reduces memorization efforts. A simple sheet of paper listing a set of *items* is a cognitive aid of this type, as well as a computer database.

The implementation of a checklist, a decision aid, a procedural document guiding the action or a memory aid has concrete consequences on the work situation, on the individual in activity (referred to as an "operator" in ergonomics). Implicitly, the presence of a cognitive aid implies a relationship with, on the one hand, an aid designer (manager, expert, ergonomist) who has deemed that assistance was necessary, defined its content, form and conditions of use and, on the other hand, an operator (doctor, nurse, aircraft pilot, etc.) who is the recipient and must apply it. This relationship is not neutral as it rests on a "helper/recipient" dynamic that places the operator-user in an asymmetrical position where part of the knowledge related to their work, part of their expertise, now depends on cognitive assistance tasked with replacing certain mental operations previously handled solely by the operator. The introduction of a checklist modifies the step of identifying the state of the world by imposing a specific order of environmental exploration and a set of objects to be identified exhaustively. A decision aid bypasses a series of arguments and calculations by directly presenting an interpretation of the situation. A to-do list provides the sequence of actions to follow, allowing for quick reference when taking action. Lastly, a memory aid avoids immediate memorization, thus enabling immediate forgetting. Therefore, to some extent, though following a similar logic of skills delegation, the introduction of a cognitive aid raises the same issue as job automation: *a device takes the place of the human operator in certain information processing tasks*.

In the realm of healthcare, the establishment of a "helper/assisted" relationship through the introduction of cognitive aid between a prescriber (the aid's designer, the manager, the expert) and an operator (the caregiver) may be perceived as atypical. Indeed, the social stereotype associated with caregivers is that of the "helper". Assisting caregivers is not an intuitive scheme. Moreover, the medical community also perpetuates the stereotype of the "knowledgeable individual". Nevertheless, through cognitive assistance, the aim is to provide them with support. This support seeks to offset a portion of their intellectual activity, which is inherently counterintuitive. Testimonials from caregivers indicate that these social representations of the caregiver and the knowledgeable individual exist both within the general populace and among healthcare professionals, for better – the anticipation of well-deserved social recognition – and for worse – the feeling of needing to embody a superhero, dedicating oneself entirely to the profession without the need for support.

These stereotypes undoubtedly account, at least partially, for the fact that it was not until the late 1990s that the concept of medical error gained recognition within institutions, becoming an operationalized concept in hospitals in a rational, almost "detached" manner, one might say. Initiating this genuine revolution in a field in which error and the notion of error-preventing aid were taboo, the hospital sector followed the trajectory set by pioneering studies in the field of aeronautics.

1.1.1. *The birth of cognitive aids: from aeronautics to the hospital sector*

On October 30, 1935, at 9:30 a.m., on the Wright Field takeoff runway in Ohio, a prototype military aircraft crashed while taking off with five crew members on board. Despite the pilot's high level of expertise – he was a test pilot – during takeoff he forgot to disengage the control that blocked the control surfaces of the aircraft, an essential component for steering the flight path. This control was one of the innovations introduced in the cockpit of the prototype aircraft 299, which would later become the B-17 Flying Fortress. Previously, the control surfaces were manually locked and unlocked on the fuselage by ground crews before takeoff.

One of the primary lessons drawn from this accident was the realization that complete reliance on the ability of pilots, even expert ones, to memorize all the intricacies of new aircraft models was not feasible. As cockpits grew in complexity, it became necessary to provide pilots with checklists enabling them to verify a set of variables before executing any critical phase of the flight (Boyne 2013). Consequently, the checklist emerged as a cognitive aid and swiftly became an indispensable component of flight procedures in military aviation (Chaparro et al. 2019).

The issue of pilots' ability to cope with increasing technological complexity gradually permeated the field of civil aviation. Indeed, the 1970s and 1980s witnessed the emergence of airliner models in which programmable logic controllers (PLCs) played an ever greater role, introducing new commands and control indicators to be assimilated by the crew. Consequently, the use of cognitive aids in cockpits naturally became imperative. During this period, civil aviation reports of flight incidents and accidents revealed that adverse events in cockpits most often pertained not to flying skills per se, but rather to peripheral skills that do not apply to the core activities for which pilots are trained. These skills, termed non-technical skills, involve operators' ability to effectively manage the resources at their disposal to address degraded situations, a concept initially referred to as cockpit resource management and later as crew resource management (CRM). Effective resource management encompasses various skills beyond basic piloting, including communication within the crew, task organization (task management), optimal team synergy (leadership and followership), appropriate decision-making based on accurate situational awareness (Endsley 1995), stress management in degraded contexts, among others. The importance of CRM in crash prevention was a key conclusion of a NASA/Industry workshop in 1979 (Lauber 1979). To optimize the assimilation of CRM best practices, the civil aviation industry will need to train pilots on flight simulators and provide them with cognitive aids.

About two decades later, the healthcare sector embraced the issue of human error and the measures to address it. A groundbreaking study on medical errors conducted across a broad spectrum of American hospitals played a pivotal role in raising this awareness. This study, documented in a 1999 report by the Institute of Medicine (IoM) (Kohn et al. 1999), became a cornerstone in the field. Its title, "To err is human", subtly reflects the stereotype of the "knowledgeable individual" being infallible, prevalent in the healthcare domain. Within this report, the authors estimated that at least 44,000 – possibly up to 98,000 – individuals died annually in the United States due to preventable medical errors. In France, since the release of the IoM report, the Ministry of Health has conducted three studies on adverse events associated with healthcare facilities (known as ENEIS): in 2004, 2009 and 2019. The latest study, ENEIS 3 (Michel et al. 2022), conducted in 2019, involved a one-week follow-up on adverse events in a sample of hospitals. This investigation revealed 123 serious adverse events (SAEs) among 4,825 patients, averaging 4.4 SAEs per 1,000 days of hospitalization, with 34% of these events deemed preventable. Comparing these figures to those from the 2009 study, the authors observed a significant decrease in preventable SAEs and their severity. However, this positive trend was not statistically significant for surgeries conducted in non-university hospital centers, critical care and implantable medical devices. The authors hypothesized that various risk management plans and programs, including the implementation of the surgical checklist introduced in France in 2010, contributed to these advancements.

A medical error, as defined in the IoM report, refers to a failure to execute an action according to the intended plan or the implementation of an inappropriate action to achieve a goal. The medical errors documented in the report encompass all facets of medical practice (Leape et al. 1993):

– the diagnostic process: diagnostic errors or delayed diagnoses, inadequate or omitted clinical examinations and failures in interpreting examination results;

– treatment: surgical, procedural or examination errors, as well as mistakes in administering medications, dosage errors, treatment delays and inappropriate care;

– preventative measures: failures in administering prophylactic treatments or monitoring treatment effects;

– additional forms of failure may include communication breakdowns, improper equipment use or other healthcare system components.

Various proposals arise from the IoM report to mitigate these risks of error. These proposals are largely inspired by practices and lessons gleaned from the aviation field. In summary, they include:

– establishing national health agencies (such as the French National Authority for Health) tasked with overseeing medical errors and providing resources to enhance the quality of care;

– implementing a reporting system for accidents and errors to learn lessons in risk management;

– standardizing care practices wherever feasible;

– organizing healthcare facilities to enhance their safety measures.

To advance this final objective, the report introduces principles grounded in an institutional-level dynamic aimed at ensuring the safety of the establishment, namely:

– facilitating respect for the limits of human capacity;

– promoting effective team functioning;

– enhancing the ability to respond to unforeseen circumstances;

– considering the establishment of a work environment conducive to learning.

Specifically, the principle of respecting human limits translates concretely into the need to design cognitive aids to surpass individuals' limited capacities, such as memory or attentional resources (vigilance), in a work setting. The caregiver is (finally) recognized as potentially vulnerable. Unfortunately, these IoM recommendations remain relevant. They still represent significant objectives for many institutions to achieve. It is noteworthy that, as in the field of aeronautics, skills beyond the core competencies in particular are acknowledged as integral to improving and ensuring the reliability of care activities.

Before the publication of this report, Dr. David Gaba, an anesthesiologist in the United States, was a pioneer in this field during the 1990s (Howard et al. 1992; Gaba et al. 1995). As an anesthetist and familiar with research in human factors and aeronautics, he observed intriguing parallels between the pilot's activity and his own work in the operating room. Both the pilot and the anesthetist are primarily tasked with continuously monitoring a process (the aircraft, the sedated patient), intervening at critical junctures (takeoff and landing, induction of and emergence from anesthesia) and managing critical incidents (technical malfunctions, anaphylactic shock in the patient). Around the same time, Rhona Flin and her team at the University of Aberdeen's Applied Psychology Laboratory in Scotland embarked on research on non-technical skills in the medical field. While David Gaba's work focused primarily on implementing CRM training sessions for anesthetists, the Aberdeen laboratory's efforts centered on developing observation grids to assess non-technical skills in simulation contexts (recorded interventions of healthcare teams on realistic mannequins). One of the initial observation grids developed was the ANTS (Anesthetists' Non-Technical Skills) framework (Fletcher et al. 2003; Flin 2013).

Since those early studies, research on human factors in the hospital setting and medical errors has surged. Gradually, hospitals have embraced these studies and their findings. One possible explanation for this enthusiasm may still lie in the image the profession can project. While the IoM report has somewhat dispelled the myth of the "superhero" caregiver, it has brought doctors closer to airline pilots, a social representation that is less idealized than that of the hero but still esteemed. Today, former airline pilots and physicians collaborate on human factors in hospitals, exchanging views and experiences to advance practices and notably to develop cognitive aids (SafetyTeam n.d.). Methods for analyzing adverse events, such as the Orion method, are being implemented (Debouck et al. 2012). Simulation has become a recommended educational method by the French National Authority for Health (*Haute Autorité de santé* or HAS) (HAS 2019), and many training programs use CRM to enhance team management of critical situations (Jaffrelot et al. 2013).

The implementation of cognitive aids in the hospital setting, inspired by the dynamics of aeronautics, has demonstrated its significance in many studies. A few examples will illustrate its extent.

1.1.2. *Contributions of cognitive aids in the medical field*

After the IoM report, numerous observations have demonstrated the value of cognitive aids in the medical field. The initial studies focused on the risks of blood infections and errors during surgery (Chaparro et al. 2019).

In 2003, a study examined methods to reduce the risk of bloodstream infections associated with catheter placement in 108 intensive care units in the state of Michigan (Pronovost et al. 2006). Following a data collection phase, a two-year intervention was conducted in these units, facilitated by remotely trained caregiver team leaders. Their role was to oversee the implementation of recommendations aimed at preventing infectious risks, including hand hygiene, precautions during central venous catheter insertion, skin preparation with chlorhexidine, avoidance of the femoral site if feasible and removal of unnecessary catheters. Alongside these practices, a checklist was introduced within the teams to ensure adherence to these recommendations. The results indicated that before the intervention, the infection rate in 55 intensive care units stood at 2.7%. During the implementation phase, it decreased to 1.6% (based on a sample of 96 services), and over the subsequent 18 months, infection rates remained at 0% per quarter (measured across 70 to 96 intensive care units). In this study, while the checklist was part of the intervention, its specific contribution to the improvement in care quality is difficult to assess, given the presence of other components such as the involvement of caregivers and training on infectious risks.

Another groundbreaking study – which centered on a checklist – is the one regarding the list of verifications to be conducted in the operating room, a cognitive aid proposed by the World Health Organization (Surgical Safety Checklist (Haynes et al. 2009)). This checklist is used across various phases of the surgical procedure: before the patient's anesthesia, before the commencement of surgery and before the patient exits the operating room (see Figure 1.2). These three intermediate moments are employed to ensure that conditions are met to proceed to the next phase in the procedure. This encompasses verifying both the patient and the surgical field (identity, localization of the operative site), the status and accessibility of equipment (operational oximeter), availability of drugs (antibiotics) and devices (patient imaging), as well as the formation of the medical team (confirmation of the entire team's presence). The items on the checklist are enumerated and verbally confirmed.

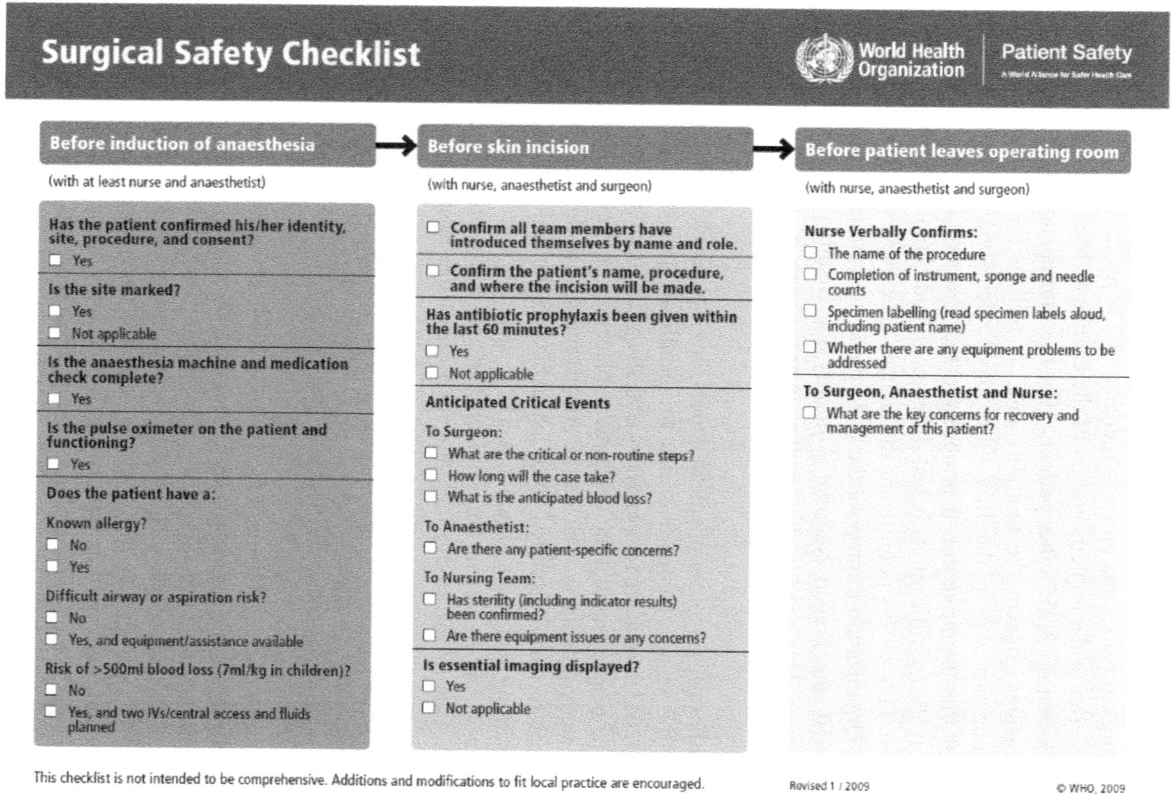

Surgical Safety Checklist

World Health Organization | Patient Safety

Before induction of anaesthesia

(with at least nurse and anaesthetist)

Has the patient confirmed his/her identity, site, procedure, and consent?
- ☐ Yes

Is the site marked?
- ☐ Yes
- ☐ Not applicable

Is the anaesthesia machine and medication check complete?
- ☐ Yes

Is the pulse oximeter on the patient and functioning?
- ☐ Yes

Does the patient have a:

Known allergy?
- ☐ No
- ☐ Yes

Difficult airway or aspiration risk?
- ☐ No
- ☐ Yes, and equipment/assistance available

Risk of >500ml blood loss (7ml/kg in children)?
- ☐ No
- ☐ Yes, and two IVs/central access and fluids planned

Before skin incision

(with nurse, anaesthetist and surgeon)

- ☐ **Confirm all team members have introduced themselves by name and role.**
- ☐ **Confirm the patient's name, procedure, and where the incision will be made.**

Has antibiotic prophylaxis been given within the last 60 minutes?
- ☐ Yes
- ☐ Not applicable

Anticipated Critical Events

To Surgeon:
- ☐ What are the critical or non-routine steps?
- ☐ How long will the case take?
- ☐ What is the anticipated blood loss?

To Anaesthetist:
- ☐ Are there any patient-specific concerns?

To Nursing Team:
- ☐ Has sterility (including indicator results) been confirmed?
- ☐ Are there equipment issues or any concerns?

Is essential imaging displayed?
- ☐ Yes
- ☐ Not applicable

Before patient leaves operating room

(with nurse, anaesthetist and surgeon)

Nurse Verbally Confirms:
- ☐ The name of the procedure
- ☐ Completion of instrument, sponge and needle counts
- ☐ Specimen labelling (read specimen labels aloud, including patient name)
- ☐ Whether there are any equipment problems to be addressed

To Surgeon, Anaesthetist and Nurse:
- ☐ What are the key concerns for recovery and management of this patient?

This checklist is not intended to be comprehensive. Additions and modifications to fit local practice are encouraged.

Revised 1 / 2009

© WHO, 2009

Figure 1.2. *Surgical Safety Checklist proposed by the World Health Organization. Reproduced with permission from WHO (2009a). For a color version of this figure, see www.iste.co.uk/morineau/cognitive.zip*

For one year (2007–2008), eight hospitals around the world – Canada, India, Jordan, New Zealand, the Philippines, Tanzania, the United Kingdom and the United States – participated in measuring the impact of this checklist on the reduction of surgical risks. Data on the surgeries of 3,733 patients over the age of 16 were collected prior to the implementation of the checklist. Then, the same types of data were collected on 3,955 other patients after the introduction of the checklist. The main measures concern the mortality rate, as well as the complication rate during hospitalization within the first thirty days after surgery. Thanks to the introduction of this cognitive aid, it is observed that the mortality rate decreased from 1.5% to 0.8% (significant statistical difference), and complications in patients decreased from 11% to 7% (significant difference). The success achieved led the World Health Organization to propose the widespread use of this checklist in 2008. In January 2010, the French National Authority for Health proposed a version adapted for France. This checklist has evolved over the years based on feedback and experience (4th version in 2018).

Recent studies using more sophisticated tools than a paper checklist, have further demonstrated the value of cognitive aids for healthcare providers. For instance, Dryver et al. (2021) conducted an experimental study employing in situ simulation (a realistic mannequin simulating the patient placed in a real emergency room setting). This study notably showcased the effectiveness of to-do lists for managing critical medical scenarios (referred to as checklists in the article, but essentially documents outlining sequences of actions). These materials were displayed on both a large screen in the treatment area and on a touchscreen tablet. Four Swedish hospitals took part in the study, including two university hospitals, one general hospital and one smaller community hospital, with the following annual emergency room visit averages: 85,000, 80,000, 65,000, 35,000. The 41 caregiver teams involved in the study comprised a total of 31 physicians (including 25 interns), 54 nurses, 37 nursing assistants and 16 medical secretaries.

Eight scenarios of critical deterioration of the patient's condition were developed (such as anaphylactic shock, severe asthma, hemorrhagic shock, septic shock, etc.). Documents outlining the necessary actions for patient management were created by an ad hoc committee of physicians for each scenario. These scenarios were conducted either with the cognitive aid disseminated on screens or without its presence. Personal cognitive aids typically used by caregivers, such as notebooks or pocket documents, were allowed, but external assistance was not permitted. A medical secretary or a nurse was trained on the dissemination procedures of the checklist and was responsible for interaction with it, without actively promoting its use to the team. Each team experienced one scenario with cognitive aid and one without. Simulation sessions were recorded and coded in double-blind fashion by emergency physicians. Four scenarios (with and without cognitive aid) were independently coded by an external physician unaware of the study's hypotheses.

This video coding enabled measurement of the percentage of checklist actions actually performed by the teams within the first fifteen minutes of patient management. The profile of the caregivers and their subjective interest in the document were also taken into account.

The results indicate no significant effect from the caregivers' profile (level of experience of doctors and nurses), as well as no effect from the presented scenarios. However, the percentage of required actions performed varies greatly between conditions with or without the checklist (see Table 1.1). With only 39% of the expected actions completed in the condition "without the checklist", the teams accomplish approximately 86% of the required actions when the checklist is present.

Without cognitive aid	With cognitive aid
38.8% [33–44%]	85.7% [80–88%]

Table 1.1. *Study by Dryver et al. (2021): median percentage of interventions performed with or without the presence of a to-do list (within the square brackets, confidence interval at p = 95%)*

The assessment of the completion of expected actions over the course of the 15-minute patient care period reveals no significant impact from the document during the initial actions. Caregivers without assistance initiate the expected actions effectively. However, after the 7th minute, the number of expected actions performed significantly increases with assistance, whereas by the 10th minute, the percentage of expected actions performed without assistance levels off at around 40%. Qualitatively, experimenters observed inappropriate or hazardous actions during the simulations. Out of the 15 risky actions observed, 14 occurred in the absence of assistance. Finally, the post-experimental questionnaire indicates that 94% of participants agreed with the statement: "I would use the checklist if I got a similar case in reality".

The authors of this study emphasize that, aside from having a document tailored to the presented medical scenario, the presence of a large screen was an essential facilitator in assisting the teams. It enabled information sharing and mutual verification of the protocol execution (cross-checking). Even though caregivers had their personal cognitive aids available in their pockets, those without on-screen assistance faced difficulties in finding practical information, such as drug dilution and administration levels. Nevertheless, two-thirds of the teams used their personal cognitive aids in the "documentless" condition.

However, two limitations are presented by the authors. Firstly, the benefit of the aid may diminish with expert doctors (the majority of doctors were interns), even though no correlation was found in this study between the doctor's experience and the team's performance. Secondly, at the beginning of the session, the medical diagnosis of the scenario was given directly to the teams. The aid only assisted in guiding patient care actions. The uncertainty associated with this critical diagnostic phase, as well as the need to navigate through numerous documents, were not dimensions evaluated by this study, dimensions that, in practice, could pose challenges.

These compelling findings have spurred significant advancements in this form of cognitive support. In France, the French National Authority for Health has thus proposed checklists for the following purposes:

– patient safety in digestive endoscopy;

– patient safety in bronchial endoscopy;

– patient safety in interventional radiology;

– placement of a central venous catheter or other vascular device;

– chemotherapy.

In 2022, the French Society of Anesthesia and Resuscitation (SFAR n.d.) offered on its website: 19 cognitive aids for crisis management in adult operating rooms, 8 for children, 6 for crisis management in delivery rooms, 14 for crisis management in intensive care units and 2 for traumatology. These aids are not exclusively checklists; some depict the medical procedure in diagram form, such as the management of an intrahospital polytraumatized patient. An increasing number of initiatives aim to provide digital platforms that offer access to a variety of cognitive aids, such as the Max platform offered by the company MEDAE[1].

A survey conducted in 2017 among doctors, nurse anesthetists and resuscitation practitioners reveals a demand for these cognitive aids among caregivers. Of the 912 respondents to the questionnaire, 94% perceive their use as enhancing care delivery during both real and simulated crisis situations, and 96% express a desire to have access to or use them more frequently (Blanié et al. 2018). However, in principle, can we reject the possibility of assistance in an intense work environment? Nonetheless, these studies demonstrate that cognitive aids serve as effective tools to support caregivers. The insights gleaned from risk management in civil aviation have proven beneficial.

1 See: https://max.medae.co/.

However, upon closer examination of the implementation details of workplace aids and their evolution over time, the conclusions to be drawn become more nuanced. The impact of cognitive aids becomes more complex, and the results vary when transitioning from concept testing in an experimental context to observing their use in real-life situations over time.

1.1.3. *Limitations in the use of medical cognitive aids*

Two studies, conducted by Gagliardi et al. (2014) and Russ et al. (2015), on the WHO Surgical Safety Checklist (SSC) highlight pitfalls that arise in the implementation of cognitive aids. The study by Gagliardi et al. (2014) involved telephone interviews with operating room caregivers in Canada, spanning small and large hospitals. In total, 29 nurses, 13 surgeons and 9 anesthesiologists were interviewed in 2011. Of these, 31 caregivers had been using the SSC in their operating rooms for a year or less, while 20 had been using it for over a year. The study by Russ et al. (2015) involved observing SSC use in five anglophone hospitals over a 13-month period, during moments of application. A total of 565 observations were conducted during surgery, and 309 observations were made at the conclusion of surgery during completion of the document.

On the one hand, the results of these two studies confirm the positive outcomes observed in other studies. Caregivers mostly express satisfaction with the contributions of the checklist. On the other hand, these studies also reveal unforeseen aspects. The usage methods vary depending on the operating rooms in hospitals. The cognitive aid can be displayed as a laminated card, a sheet of paper, or a wall poster. These variable usage modalities alter how team members access the content of the checklist. Depending on the format, this may involve listening to the caregiver listing the items or visual access for everyone. It is noteworthy that there are no established rules justifying one presentation mode over another. Furthermore, it was observed that most caregivers interviewed admitted to modifying the checklist proposed to them, sometimes significantly. In its original form, it did not meet their requirements. In certain instances, different versions are combined to create an entirely new checklist. These adaptations are motivated by the need to tailor it to the specific practices of an operating room, such as defining each individual's roles in completing the cognitive aid or determining when each item should be addressed.

In a more critical light, it is observed that the use of cognitive aids can sometimes be unsystematic or incomplete. In the study by Gagliardi et al. (2014), most participants reported that the SSC room checklist is either read incompletely or not used systematically. Russ et al. (2014) noted that essential information such as the patient's identity and procedure identification, which are crucial in the checklist, are absent in 10% of the observed cases. Furthermore, the involvement of all team members in checkpoints with the checklist is not consistent. Russ et al. (2014) observed that some team members are absent during the verification phase in over 40% of cases. Even when present, they often fail to focus their attention on completing the checklist in more than 70% of cases. During the final stage of the surgical procedure, verification is omitted in 39% of the observed procedures, reaching up to 87% in one of the hospitals sampled. Frequently, the surgeon is no longer present during this final phase. The issue arises when the final phase checklist is completed earlier, often leading to neglect of the part concerning the nurse, highlighting the team's difficulty in considering the final verification as an integral component of the surgical procedure. In some instances, Gagliardi et al. (2014) reported that even when the cognitive aid items were systematically reviewed within the team, the staff either engaged in unrelated conversations or simply disregarded them. To them, it appeared as a mere "routine", "additional checkboxes to check". Sometimes, it is documented that the SSC was used in the report, although it was not the case in reality.

These modifications in the terms of use, as well as the actual content used, demonstrate a process of re-appropriation, and sometimes non-appropriation, of the document. Caregivers go beyond mere implementation; they actively redefine the methods of use and the content of cognitive aids. On the non-appropriation side, reactions can present real obstacles to effective use of cognitive aids. Operators may perceive the documents as irrelevant to their activities. Some may view the existing organization of their work as incompatible with the introduction of a checklist. The introduction of new pause stages to complete it may be seen as disrupting the necessary flow required for critical patient management tasks. Introducing a new device could be perceived as an interruption in an activity flow already frequently disrupted by daily interruptions or an additional administrative layer whose function duplicates other checklists and checkpoints.

Individual queries can also impede adoption, stemming from uncertainty regarding the efficacy of such a document, and the prescribed conditions of use (when, how, by whom). The absence of evidence presented to staff regarding the effectiveness of the checklist further amplifies this uncertainty. A verification process involving the entire team, but singling out a specific caregiver tasked with listing the items to be verified, can disrupt the structure of a team accustomed to traditional hierarchical dynamics typically led by the physician. When a nurse assumes the role of verifying the state of affairs, it may be perceived as encroaching on established authority. Moreover, cognitive aids may be perceived as challenging the expertise of the staff, knowledge founded on years of rigorous study and daily practice. This becomes evident when considering that a cognitive aid, through its functions, assumes responsibility for certain steps of information processing originally within the scope of one or more individuals in the team.

These reactions can be intensified by a failure to consider the perspective of future cognitive aid users by managers during the implementation of the device. As with any new tool introduced into the array of resources available to operators, change management must be implemented. This involves actions such as the following:

– *Dissemination of information regarding the expected benefits of cognitive aid*: Gagliardi et al. (2014) occasionally observes that teams are informed solely via email or memorandum about the introduction of the checklist.

– *A definition of the conditions for using the checklist, and even collaborative development of its content in a co-design approach*: many caregivers in both studies reported feeling that the checklist was imposed on them by managers, which sometimes affected morale in the operating room and caused tensions.

– *A testing and training phase is necessary for the teams to effectively adopt the device:* in one of the studies, nurses, who were largely responsible for planning the implementation of the SSC, reported having had little time to test it before its final launch.

– *Monitoring the implementation of the device:* the adoption of such a device unfolds over time. "Relay" caregivers serving as references must be identified to ensure the sustainability of the action. Monitoring its use is essential to identify adherence problems and implement necessary modifications. However, only a few sites in the two cited studies conducted follow-ups on usage through periodic data collection. There appeared to be no encouragement for using the checklist nor a clear definition of the consequences associated with non-adherence.

It can be hypothesized that these shortcomings during the introduction of cognitive aids are linked to an overly simplistic definition of such aids. This simplifying definition assumes that cognitive aids are inherently helpful, given their purpose and content, and thus do not require upfront justification and testing. Following this logic, there is no need for an appropriation process. However, this perspective on cognitive aids overlooks the viewpoint of users in real-life situations. In practice, cognitive aids are trivially perceived by users as technical-administrative devices among others, which integrate into usual operating methods and inevitably alter the balance in the work situation and the constraints to be respected.

If we wish to consider the "user" viewpoint, it is essential to acknowledge the inevitable process of appropriation. To ensure successful appropriation, it is necessary to focus on two well-known criteria in ergonomics: usefulness and ease of use of the implemented device. The caregiver, like any other operator, does not passively receive a working document intended as an aid; rather, they actively integrate it, in varying degrees of ease and completeness, into their daily activities, depending on the document's utility and user-friendliness. This leads us to a new perspective defining cognitive aid, modestly, as a simple instrument in operators' toolkit.

1.2. Cognitive aid defined as an instrument

The SFAR defines a *cognitive aid as "a tool created to guide its user in the performance of one or more tasks"* (Bijok et al. 2022, p. 9). The concept of a tool is crucial, representing a functional means of intervention in reality. Here, we adopt the term "instrument" to better integrate the notion of a psychological instrument. Three elements justify defining a cognitive aid primarily as an instrument.

The first argument lies in the necessity of having a more neutral definition, less oriented than one based on the idea that cognitive aids compensate for potential failures in operators' reasoning. By defining cognitive aids as devices that support mental activity, there is a risk of focusing on human vulnerabilities, which could be a source of errors. Implicitly, this leads to the conclusion that the origin of a failure in information processing is likely to be a lack of ability or skills in the human operator. While the level of expertise is undoubtedly a potential factor explaining a failure in the chain of reasoning, *cognitive aids primarily serve as a means to mitigate the effects of work situations on cognition (such as unusual situations, stress, high time pressure, high workload, etc.) rather than compensating for operators' skills*. In aiming to improve working conditions through cognitive aids, the central element to consider is that work contexts that generate excessive mental load are a major source of error. These contexts must be made more reliable through the use of cognitive aids.

The second element is that *nothing prohibits a cognitive aid from being a means to enhance information processing capacities beyond expectations*. It is not necessarily a way to compensate for cognitive fragility in a given context. A cognitive aid is not a cognitive prosthesis; rather, it can enable improved performance beyond merely maintaining stability in degraded working conditions, much like any ordinary tool that enhances the ability to act on the environment.

Finally, when we aim to comprehensively define cognitive aids, considering whether a particular device belongs to the cognitive aids category or not, we observe that *many work instruments can ultimately fulfill the role of cognitive aid*. Let us revisit the information processing chain proposed by Rasmussen. The identification phase of the situation can be supported, as previously mentioned, by checklists that facilitate verification of the state of the world and/or the effects of actions taken. But what about an alarm on a physiological monitor? Is this not assisting in detecting information about the patient's condition? If alarms are considered cognitive aids, then this also encompasses many information systems that transmit alert messages. In the decision-making phase, a chart aids in interpreting a situation by, for instance, providing the expected weight of a child for a given age. Additionally, an artificial intelligence program capable of interpreting a medical image contributes to decision-making. In the action planning phase, beyond documents that describe work procedures, schedules or action plans assist in sequencing actions over time, like the speech synthesis integrated into a defibrillator guiding the rescuer's actions. Similarly, a "patient" file serves as a device for storing information, reducing memorization efforts and thus aiding in memorization across various stages of information processing. More broadly, a simple information system comprising a piece of paper and a pencil constitutes a cognitive aid. Just like a shopping list, the half-sheet of paper and the pencil used by a doctor in an emergency department to take notes on patients support cognitive activity as an easy-to-use memory aid, tailored to the user's needs and designed by the user themselves (see Figures 1.3 and 1.4).

Considering cognitive aids as part of the broader category of instruments offers a distinct advantage. It enables their integration into the customary process of instrument design, a well-established practice among engineers and ergonomists. This design process incorporates the necessity of considering users' perspectives and assessing their functional requirements. Like any standard instrument, a cognitive aid must adhere to two major ergonomic criteria to meet the functional needs of operators: *utility* and *ease of use (also known as "usability").*

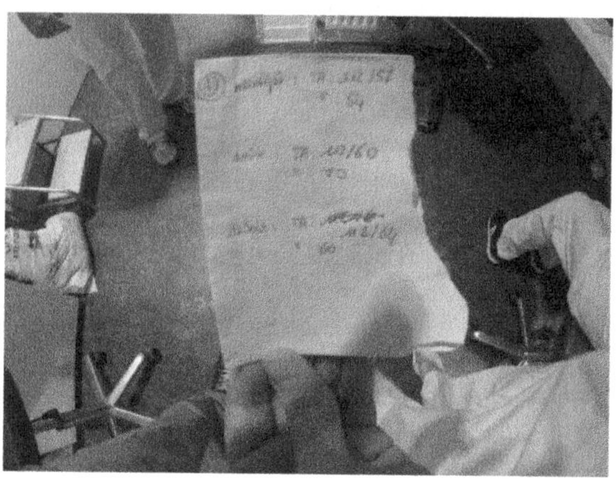

Figure 1.3. *Cognitive aid in the pocket of a medical resident in an emergency department (photo credit: T. Morineau)*

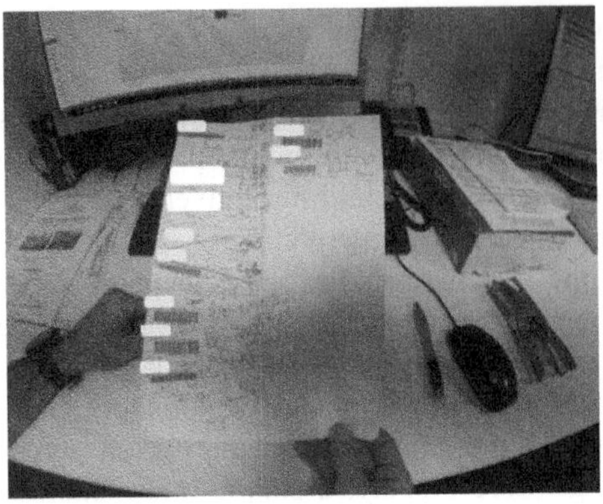

Figure 1.4. *Cognitive aid in the pocket of a senior physician in an emergency department (photo credit: T. Morineau)*

1.2.1. *Utility of the cognitive aid*

To consider that a cognitive aid inherently brings benefits to its users is a simplistic view. It fails to address how the device will be received by its users and the actual impact it may have in real-life situations, whether positive or negative. Introducing an instrument that has not undergone a thorough design process, including an analysis of the real activity of the intended operators, involves significant risks. Even a device assumed to be inherently helpful can disrupt and degrade the flow of activity, upsetting the balance within the work system. Previous descriptions of the use of the operating room block checklist illustrate this point.

The existence of cognitive aids developed by their own users underscores the significance of the utility criterion in the emergence of assistive devices. This demonstrates that these ad hoc solutions fundamentally address a need in information processing. In this context, the operator creates their own assistance using the available resources, which is somewhat paradoxical when considering the strict definition of cognitive aid as a device provided by an external agent to assist operators in difficulty. Moreover, the creation of cognitive aids for oneself indicates that the user of assistance is not a passive agent awaiting help. Instead, they have the capacity to become a designer themselves during their use of instruments. They can delegate some of their cognitive skills to an external device. A portion of the information stored in memory is intentionally transferred to a piece of paper kept in the pocket of a gown.

During the process of designing a cognitive aid, the utility criterion of the device must be examined through an analysis of the work of the operators concerned. This analysis will allow us to consider how the cognitive aid can be integrated into the activity by providing real benefits in terms of performance, risk reduction and operator comfort at work. To assess the utility of a cognitive aid, it is also necessary to consider the operators' levels of expertise in this work analysis. A cognitive aid may be beneficial for novice operators but unnecessary for experts. The fact that experts do not use it does not necessarily indicate a partial failure of the intervention; rather, it suggests that the aid has been appropriately targeted to specific functions. In principle, it is advisable to reject assistance if it proves to be unnecessary given the demands of the work context and the operators' ability to manage it, at least at some point during the activity.

1.2.2. *Ease of use of the cognitive aid*

Once again, contrary to the idea that a cognitive aid would inherently provide assistance, its introduction can introduce additional constraints due to a lack of consideration for the actual conditions of use. Many have had experience with instruments or devices deemed fundamentally useful but difficult to use or comprehend due to ergonomic shortcomings. Numerous working documents prove challenging to read due to excessive length, small font sizes or confusing structures, such as poorly designed diagrams or disorganized layouts.

A classic example of neglecting ease of use is attempting to include all the information from the instructions or recommendations described in the original texts. By exhaustively transcribing the requirements, the document becomes unreadable in a work environment where caregivers are inundated with multiple sources of information and time constraints. For instance, a medical device manufacturer once tasked a student during an internship to improve the usability and ergonomics of a user guide for the medical equipment it sold. With over a hundred pages, this document was simply unreadable and consequently stored away in cabinets without ever being consulted. In reality, the company viewed this document not only as a user manual but also as a legally binding text. By outlining all the risks associated with device misuse, they were legally safeguarding themselves. The criterion of ease of use was sacrificed in favor of another function assigned to the document.

Viewing cognitive aids as instruments introduces the need for a genuine "user-oriented" design process, integrating an understanding of the requirements of working conditions to ensure the device is genuinely useful and usable. However, this instrumental perspective has its limitations. Indeed, embedding cognitive aids within the broad spectrum of human instruments no longer allows for sufficient precision in defining them clearly from other ordinary instruments found in a work environment. While cognitive aids are indeed instruments, they are distinct instruments: they serve as cognitive gateways.

1.3. Gateway function

We will argue that the purpose of a cognitive aid is to serve as a gateway facilitating the routing of cognitive resources, thereby assisting the operator in carrying out one or more tasks[2].

If we refer to the Cambridge dictionary definition, a "gateway" is described as "a place through which you have to go to get to another place". Such a gateway facilitates the crossing of obstacles, enabling transit that would otherwise be difficult or impossible. A gateway serves as a means of routing resources between two points, allowing movement in both directions. To delve deeper into this metaphor, we could describe *a cognitive aid as a supplementary device that supports task execution by facilitating the routing of resources for information processing, including knowledge and reasoning capabilities.* Expanding on this metaphor, a cognitive gateway can be likened to a portable tool, capable of being relocated and positioned in various locations to facilitate movement from one point to another. This versatility allows for different starting and ending points in the routing of cognitive resources.

The surrounding environment can serve as the initial destination. Through a gateway positioned between an environment and an individual, the individual allocates a portion of their cognitive resources to the environment, where they will remain stored for a certain period of time. Writing a shopping list on a piece of paper represents this transfer of information to an external device (the piece of paper). In the case of a checklist, providing it to operators as a working document signifies the transfer of a verification task to an external device (the checklist). Then, at the appropriate moment, these resources will revert, returning to the individual's cognition to support their cognitive activity. The shopping list will be consulted while browsing store aisles. The checklist will be used by the operator during a verification phase.

2 A task is defined as "a specified goal under predetermined conditions" (Leplat and Hoc 1983). This goal can be assigned by a supervisor or initiated by the individual themselves. The conditions encompass various aspects including physical, organizational, social and functional factors.

However, within the internal cognitive mechanisms themselves, there are possibilities for back-and-forth movements between different cognitive locations, facilitated by cognitive gateways. The operator can thus channel resources from their capacity to reason analytically or from their intuitive thinking. Through these pathways, they provide responses that navigate obstacles and vulnerabilities in information processing. For instance, based on acquired experience, it is possible to intuitively estimate the weight of a child relative to their age and physical appearance, aiding in determining the dosage of a medication to be administered. Furthermore, using a precise and reliable measurement from a scale offers another approach to accomplishing the same task, this time by accessing analytical resources. In this scenario, the scale acts as a cognitive gateway. Other aids also enable the reverse journey, channeling intuitive resources to facilitate quick and effortless decision-making.

Another form of transit facilitated by a cognitive gateway is the transfer of prescriptions from experts in a domain or managers to the operator (the caregiver) engaged in activity and in need of these prescriptions at a given moment. A cognitive gateway serves to bridge the gap between the expectations regarding best practices from the prescribers of such practices and the diverse and variable constraints encountered in actual caregiving activity. Documents outlining medical directives exemplify a gateway aimed at routing expert knowledge to caregivers.

However, irrespective of the "locations" a cognitive gateway aims to connect, users must have complete confidence in it as an efficient means of obtaining cognitive reinforcement. A cognitive gateway must also be reliable and easily accessible during its implementation. Any transfer of cognitive resources should be executed with minimal effort and with evident benefits, to avoid posing an additional constraint on the activity.

2

Cognitive Aid: A Gateway Between the Individual and their Environment

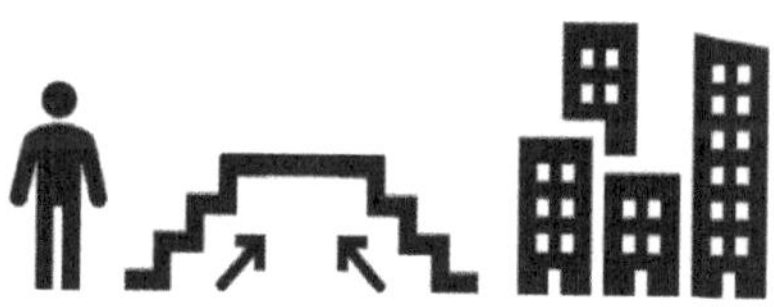

Figure 2.1. *Cognitive aid as a bidirectional gateway between the individual and their environment*

One of the major concerns regarding cognitive aids is the potential loss of skills among their users, as certain mental operations and knowledge are taken over by external devices. This concern extends far beyond the hospital setting; it applies to all situations, which are becoming increasingly common, whereby an artificial information processing system handles certain tasks at work, in learning contexts, or in everyday life. These tasks may involve identification, participation in decision-making, action guidance, writing or memorization, as per our previous classification of cognitive aids.

By delegating arithmetic calculations to a calculator, does a middle school student not risk losing their competence in mental calculation? While a calculator helps avoid laborious and repetitive calculations, it also diminishes opportunities to engage internal skills, thereby gradually weakening them. Multiplication tables may gradually fade from memory, at least in part.

A crucial skill in humans, as in any animal, for everyday adaptation is spatial orientation. With the increasing reliance on GPS assistance, are we at risk of losing our visuo-spatial ability to represent and orient ourselves in space? A study involving 24 participants, navigating the Soho district of London using GPS, revealed that brain regions responsible for spatial orientation (the hippocampus linked with prefrontal areas) were "deactivated" during GPS use (Javadi et al. 2017). The researchers concluded that frequent GPS usage could potentially harm our long-term spatial orientation ability.

In antiquity, Plato lamented the advent of writing, a technique that supplanted the memorization skills of young learners. It is noteworthy that the *Iliad* and the *Odyssey* were originally transmitted orally in songs rather than chapters, demanding significant memorization efforts. Today, vast Internet databases grant access to vast amounts of precise knowledge in a few clicks, negating the need for memorization. Will encyclopedic-type knowledge storage in the human brain remain necessary in the future? Just as robots now replace human operators in manual tasks, software also generates content without human intervention. As artificial intelligence develops, intellectual activity is increasingly automated. Any cognitive aid represents the initial stages of knowledge automation. A simple list marks the beginning of knowledge formalization. By further modeling this process, a flowchart could be generated, potentially leading to a logical algorithm designed for software to manage the listed tasks. For instance, one of the earliest artificial intelligence programming languages, LISP (list processing), is based on simple logical sequences of symbol lists. Therefore, concerns about the gradual replacement of certain cognitive activities by automatic systems, such as those in generative artificial intelligence currently in development, are indeed warranted.

However, beneath these concerns stemming from artificial intelligence or robotics, research in the field of human factors has demonstrated that complete automation of a workstation is often more of an automation engineer's ideal than a reality. Industries that were early adopters of extensive automation plans, such as aviation, steel production or nuclear power, have shown that humans do not vanish from the workplace but rather adopt different roles. Traditionally, the operator transitions from executing the action (operator) to overseeing it, a task now performed by an automated system (supervisor). A common example is seen in the role of cashiers in supermarkets. While some checkout processes have been automated, they still require a supervisor to assist customers encountering difficulties and to troubleshoot malfunctioning systems.

The function of a supervisor does not resolve the issue of expertise loss associated with automation. Sectors that have undergone significant automation have demonstrated that the risk of skill loss exists among supervisors as well. When automation systems experience technical failures, the operation must switch to manual mode, requiring supervisors to regain control and resume operator duties. This represents a critical phase that necessitates the reactivation of latent knowledge. Simulation exercises simulating degraded situations can help compensate for this loss by reactivating dormant knowledge. In the context of healthcare, professionals currently use simulation to maintain skills that are used infrequently. Perhaps, one day, healthcare providers transitioning into healthcare process supervisors will make use of simulation to reacquire proficiency in manual operations.

Regardless, given that a new cognitive aid introduces a form of automation, however rudimentary, it is crucial to consider this aspect during the design of a new work aid. However, this aspect will remain problematic if the problem analysis focuses solely on the effects of devices on internal cognition. In other words, without considering the overall cognitive system and its dynamics, which comprises not only the operator (the caregiver) but also the ambient environment that can support knowledge.

2.1. The cognitive system: knowledge in the head and in the environment

The issue of knowledge loss due to artificial information processing systems is a poorly formulated problem. It centers on the individual and the internal cognitive resources they may lose. In this context, the concern is how much of the operator's own resources can be withdrawn and outsourced to artificial systems, and which resources should be automated. The primary criterion for decision-making becomes performance: tasks in which artificial devices outperform humans should be delegated to the devices, while those better handled by humans should remain their responsibility (Fitts 1951). As technology advances in artificial intelligence, humans and machines are seen as being in constant competition for cognitive skills, leading to a pessimistic outlook: humans are likely to eventually lose the competition without benefiting from technological progress unless they are viewed in a trans-humanist perspective, as cyborgs implanted with processors and nanomachines.

However, if the approach to the problem shifts away from focusing solely on the individual and the knowledge losses caused by artificial devices, a different perspective emerges. An alternative viewpoint is to regard the individual and their surrounding environment – which includes artificial information processing devices – as a unified entity, a global cognitive system. Within this system, both the individual and their environment can possess cognitive resources, and these resources can be transferred between different components of the system. The crucial performance metric then becomes that of the overall system rather than the performance of any single component. For instance, while software may be highly efficient on its own, its lack of ergonomics can lead to poor user performance, thereby compromising the effectiveness of the overall human–machine system. Conversely, operators' expertise may not translate into good performance if they rely on inefficient or faulty technical devices. With this realization, *the location of knowledge becomes less important; what matters is whether the global cognitive system is capable of achieving a set of objectives.*

In their article *"The extended mind"*, Clark and Chalmers (1998) initiate their inquiry with the question: "Where does the mind stop and where does the rest of the world begin?". They propose two distinct answers to this question. The first, a more traditional view, suggests that what lies outside the body is beyond the realm of the mind. Knowledge is conceptualized as an abstract entity residing within individuals' minds. Conversely, the second approach underscores the involvement of the environment in shaping knowledge. Fundamentally, the meaning of words is not confined to individuals' minds but is rooted in the world that serves as a reference point and to which the thinking individual belongs. Moreover, humans, through their symbolic abilities, continuously generate – having done so since the dawn of time – symbols that permeate their living environment, influencing their thought processes. Therefore, cognition is not solely confined to the mind but is also intertwined with the environment. This externalist perspective characterizes the latter view of cognition.

In an externalist approach, the relevant unit of analysis is the "environment–individual" system, which the American psychologist John Dewey (1859–1952) more simply referred to as "the situation". We cannot comprehend an individual's mental activity without considering their surrounding environment, where signs are both read and written. Conversely, understanding this environment requires viewing it through the perspective of its users and how it is used. Clark and Chalmers (1998) illustrate this with a mental rotation exercise similar to Tetris (the well-known video game). This playful task involves constructing a uniform wall by rotating variously shaped pieces on the screen to fit them together horizontally. Originally, this game was played on a computer, with the player rotating pieces using keyboard arrows. However, the same task could be accomplished solely by a player mentally visualizing and rotating the pieces (dedicated Tetris players could attest to this ability, often seeing pieces fall even after closing their eyes post-game). Looking ahead, we might envision implanting a processor in the player's brain, triggered at will to execute the necessary rotations. These three information processing configurations extend to other tasks, such as chess; some players can play, and even win, blindfolded. These three configurations show that the same cognitive task can be performed with a highly variable distribution of resources without considering bodily limitations. In the first case, resources are divided between the external environment and the player. In the second case, these resources are solely within the player who imagines performing the task. In the third case, the human loses some of their contribution by delegating certain mental operations to a neural implant. In purely functional terms and on the scale of the overall "individual–environment" system encompassing the technical device (computer or neural implant) and the player, the three configurations lead to the same result: the production of a performance assessable by the same criteria such as speed or success rate. The quality of this performance will depend on the efficiency of the chosen configuration.

The second example provided by Clark and Chalmers (1998) brings us closer to understanding cognitive aids. This hypothetical scenario involves two individuals, Inga and Otto. Inga, wanting to attend an exhibition, mentally recalls the precise address of the museum before leaving. On the contrary, Otto, who suffers from Alzheimer's disease, uses a notebook daily that contains key information, including the museum's address, as he cannot rely on his memory.

If we analyze these situations focusing solely on individuals and excluding their surrounding environment, the cognitive impairment resulting from Otto's illness becomes prominent. However, if we consider the global cognitive system encompassing both the individual and the environment, then we can argue that the two scenarios are functionally comparable. Both visitors will be able to reach the museum by retrieving the address from either internal memory or external memory. The difference, once again, lies in the allocation of cognitive resources between the individual and their environment to accomplish the task.

According to Clark and Chalmers (1998), the distribution of cognitive resources between the individual and their environment within a cognitive system is inconsequential. *What truly matters is the dynamic nature of exchanges between the individual and their environment, facilitating the seamless transfer of knowledge from one point to another. Clark and Chalmers identify three primary criteria – trust, reliability and accessibility – for ensuring high-quality exchanges within such systems.* These criteria apply not only to the information content stored within cognitive resources but also to the mediums used for storage (see Table 2.1). Consequently, the effectiveness of interactions, whether between Otto and his notebook or Inga and her long-term memory, hinges on the fulfillment of these three criteria.

	Information content	**Information tool**
Trust	Confidence in the source of information	Confidence in the utility of the tool
Reliability	Quality of information (updating)	Risk of failure of the tool
Accessibility	Ease of reading and understanding	Ease of use of the tool

Table 2.1. *Criteria for evaluating the qualities of a cognitive aid in terms of its content and tool*

The contribution of each component of a cognitive system (the environment and the human component) can evolve over time, as well as according to contexts. For example, let us imagine that unfortunately Otto's condition deteriorates, his disease is progressing; then the environment must play an increased role in achieving a number of daily objectives: the notebook at the bottom of his pocket may transform into a table at his home, partially filled in by his relatives or with the support of a home aide. If, by chance, Otto's condition improves, simply taking notes in his notebook may suffice to remember them without needing to reread them. Many individuals take notes without ever revisiting them, yet this single action facilitates assimilation of information during the writing process.

Furthermore, in a very prosaic manner, considering the cognitive system as composed of both the individual and their environment, rather than solely the individual delimited by their body, helps to alleviate the guilt of cognitive aid users who fear being judged as incompetent. For example, individuals may consult the Vidal for precise medication characteristics or refer to their memory aid for dosages in pediatric preparations (the stereotype of the "knowing" individual). From prehistoric cave paintings to the "fully digital" age in which mobile phones are integrated into daily life for some, including the invention of the printing press, humans have always inscribed symbols in their environment to preserve information over time and facilitate its sharing within a collective. *Just because a cognitive aid is inherently external does not mean it should be avoided, but rather because its access is not certain, it is less reliable, less accessible and less trusted in its ability to support goal attainment, compared to another external or internal means that provides the same function*. Users of a calculator may have greater confidence in arriving at the correct result of a complex calculation using this instrument rather than relying on mental calculation. They can also rely on the reliability of this well-established technology. However, they may question the accessibility of the calculator in all situations. On this last criterion, mental calculation may prevail in the comparison, which implies long-term efforts to preserve this cognitive skill. If the goal is to acquire calculation skills, then confidence will lean more towards individual mental work than the use of a calculator. Nonetheless, learners can use the calculator to verify that mental calculations are correct (the do-confirm approach, a mode of using cognitive aids that can be relevant as we will see later). Paradoxically, in this example, the calculator has become a tool for the internalization of knowledge. In other words, for a young student, learning multiplication tables does not mean abstaining from using the calculator. Rather, it involves defining an operational mode of using this instrument to support the internalization of skills. Research on learning has shown that asking students to solve mathematical problems while simultaneously providing the solution results in better learning of the underlying mathematical concepts, compared to a situation in which they had to solve these problems without this aid (Sweller and Cooper 1985; Puma and Tricot 2021). This means that even in a learning context aimed explicitly at acquiring new internal knowledge, an external cognitive aid (the presentation of the problem solution) facilitates the effort of internalizing knowledge. This counterintuitive result contradicts a static description of knowledge distribution, with some knowledge stored in the environment and the remainder stored in the individual. If information processing by the individual is dynamic and active, then a synergy between knowledge inscribed in the environment and that in the brain will occur. In short, by analyzing real-life use situations of external resources as dynamic systems, it is possible to observe more complex exchanges between internal cognition and external cognition than mere knowledge storage in external devices that replace humans.

These considerations shed light on the fact that, like any typical tool, artificial information processing systems have the potential to significantly enhance cognitive capabilities. External assistance and internal cognition interact synergistically, enriching the mental activities of individuals within such systems. In the same way that humans have developed mechanical technologies to increase their influence on the environment, their history is characterized by cognitive technologies that have expanded their capacity to process information. These technologies, termed "psychological instruments" by psychologist Lev Vygotsky (1896–1934), normalize the use of cognitive aids in human activities and suggest that such aids can enhance cognition by promoting greater thought organization among users. As posited by a systemic approach, the entirety of a cognitive system, encompassing both individual and environmental components, surpasses the sum of its parts.

2.2. Cognitive aid as a psychological instrument

A psychological instrument resembles and simultaneously distinguishes itself from an ordinary tool. Like the latter, it serves as an intermediary for carrying out an action. For instance, a saw is an ordinary tool used to manipulate materials. Conversely, language, considered a psychological instrument by Vygotsky, enables individuals to influence both themselves and others through communication. Furthermore, both types of instruments are deeply intertwined with cultural and social contexts. They represent human constructs that can be transmitted socially and are shaped by the experiences of preceding generations, who refined the characteristics of tools like the saw or the linguistic features of a language reflective of a particular culture.

While an ordinary instrument acts on nature, a psychological instrument operates on the psyche. *Unlike an ordinary instrument, a psychological instrument is primarily a system of signs designed to control one's own cognition or that of others*. According to Vygotsky, a sign is "any artificial stimulus created by individuals as a means of controlling their own behavior or that of others" (Schneuwly 1987). Numerous psychological instruments can be identified. Vygotsky lists "language, various forms of counting and calculation, mnemonic devices, algebraic symbols, works of art, writing, diagrams, charts, maps, plans, all possible signs, etc." (Friedrich 2012). All of these instruments share the characteristic of being sign structures capable of facilitating the flow of thought. It is worth noting that mnemonic devices, diagrams, charts, maps and plans can easily be classified as cognitive aids. However, not all psychological instruments are inherently cognitive aids. For example, language serves a much broader psychological function. Language, extensively studied by Vygotsky (2012), is not simply a cognitive aid. A child acquiring language does not perceive this activity as an aid to reasoning or memorization. Language, like drawing or graphic representation, serves as a natural means to share individual thoughts within a collective, to access shared knowledge and to gain a deeper understanding of the world. Secondly, language supports thought by providing a means to enhance its structuring. Additionally, while language is indeed a system of artificial signs, it has not been subject, strictly speaking, to a design process at a given moment, as a cognitive aid might be. Therefore, cognitive aids are a specific type of psychological instrument (Figure 2.2). Cognitive aids are intentionally designed devices created within a specific space-time to assist in processing information in particular situations in which specific cognitive tasks need to be performed. These are instruments dedicated to a group of workers or an individual (such as taking notes on a piece of paper) and are subject to modification within a relatively short timeframe, such as updating workplace best practices, or may even be discarded after completing the task (such as notes in a gown pocket).

The primary objective of a cognitive aid is to *facilitate the structuring of thought*, while incidentally conveying knowledge that is socially and culturally embedded. For instance, while a medical encyclopedia serves as a psychological instrument aimed at transmitting shared knowledge within a profession at a specific time, the surgical checklist functions as a cognitive aid primarily assisting the team in crucial aspects of their activity during the short period of a surgery. However, there exists a continuous connection between general psychological instruments and specific cognitive aids. An example illustrating this continuum is the vortex metaphor employed to address patient oxygenation in emergency medicine (Chrimes 2016).

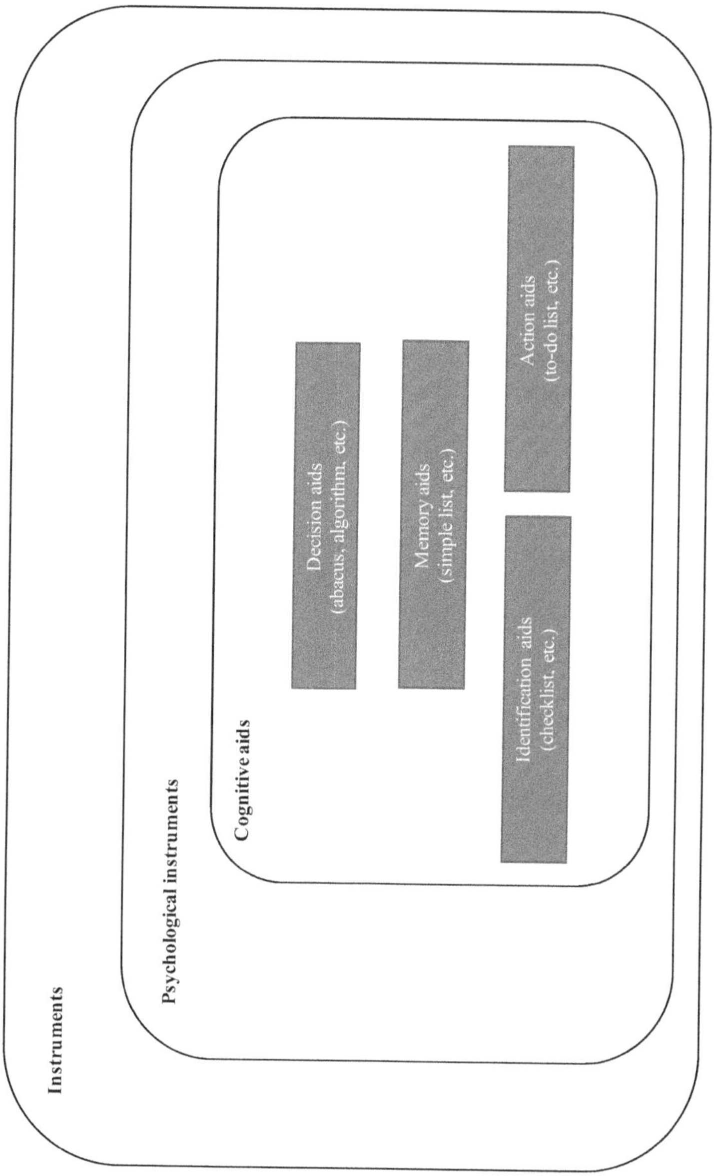

Figure 2.2. *Cognitive aids: subset of psychological instruments and instruments in general*

2.2.1. *The vortex in emergency medicine*

The cognitive aid known as the "vortex" targets a critical phase in patient resuscitation, specifically the provision of oxygenation. Chrimes (2016) has devised a metaphorical language through the vortex to facilitate the execution of this sequence of critical care. Drawing from the concept of ergonomist Pierre Falzon (1987), a genuine operative language has been crafted, comprising professional jargon tailored to the operational requirements arising from the activity.

2.2.1.1. *The semantics of the vortex*

To facilitate easy access to knowledge and skills in managing oxygenation, the vortex serves as a metaphor. A vortex resembles a funnel-shaped whirlpool. This analogy draws a parallel between a complex domain and a more accessible representation. The vortex metaphor illustrates the progression to follow in implementing oxygenation techniques.

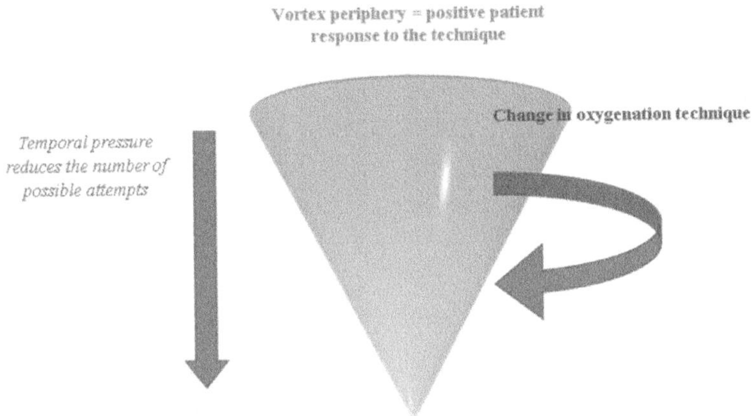

Figure 2.3. *The vortex analogy to describe the progression in the oxygenation procedure of a patient. Figure inspired by Chrimes (2016) and Vortex Approach (n.d.). For a color version of this figure, see www.iste.co.uk/morineau/cognitive.zip*

Figure 2.3 is inspired by one of the representations provided to teams to grasp the logic of the vortex. At the periphery of the vortex, depicted in green, the patient is breathing effectively. Entry into the core of the vortex (outside the periphery) indicates that caregivers are faced with the need to oxygenate the patient. As the physician attempts techniques that prove unsuccessful (oxygen mask, laryngeal mask, intubation, tracheotomy), they are drawn downwards into the vortex, corresponding to a progressive reduction in ventilation solutions, with the patient's respiratory condition becoming increasingly critical. In this deteriorating dynamic, the situation demands the use of increasingly invasive techniques, ultimately leading to a tracheotomy, i.e. a surgical opening for direct access to the trachea. It is noteworthy that unlike a flowchart typically used to describe such medical protocols, entry into the vortex can occur from any point by choosing a technique deemed most suitable for the patient, and depending on the patient's condition. Furthermore, each member of the healthcare team can symbolically be located at different points in the vortex, with the nurse preparing the next technique while the physician attempts the initial one. Beyond the figure presented here, a set of illustrated figures is given to teams to understand the vortex logic. For instance, a reminder of key elements applicable to any technique is presented: patient manipulation to clear the airways, equipment preparation, assistance call, selection of appropriate equipment size and type (mask size, tube size, etc.), airway suction if necessary, oxygen flow rate selection, muscle tone verification, etc.

This original description allows for consideration of the specificities of patient resuscitation in emergency situations, including a dynamic progression (in relation to trials and time pressure), parallel progression (various roles within the team during the procedure) and potentially cyclical progression (returning to less invasive phases if the patient's condition improves). These aspects of real-world activity are challenging to depict accurately with a traditional flowchart based on a linear sequence.

2.2.1.2. *The lexicon of the vortex*

However, the contributions of this cognitive aid extend beyond a mere display. The analogy used has broader scope, becoming a general way of understanding oxygenation and a new reference point during communication within the team. Firstly, the poster describing the vortex relies on a standardized lexicon, composed of symbols representing different oxygenation techniques and keywords recalling key elements in the implementation of a technique. More importantly, terminology associated with the cognitive aid is provided. For instance, the authors propose the phrase "being in the green zone" to express that the patient has regained sufficient oxygen saturation, or "being drawn into the vortex" when time passes and the number of oxygenation solutions is reduced. This metaphorical lexicon aims to facilitate the sharing of situational awareness among caregivers. The use of such a lexicon helps to structure verbal exchanges.

2.2.1.3. *Objects referring to the vortex*

Linguist Ferdinand de Saussure delineated the structure of language as grounded in signifieds (semantics, the meaning attributed to words), signifiers (lexicon) and referents (the real-world objects to which signifiers and signifieds correspond). We have just examined the signifieds (the oxygenation procedure and its metaphor) and the signifiers (the lexicon of the vortex) of the cognitive aid. Additionally, this aid also refers to tangible objects in the care environment. For instance, an emergency cart has been designed to organize medical instruments according to the logic of the vortex, using colors, symbols and the structured presentation of oxygenation phases in communication tools. This approach solidifies the procedural description logic by physically embedding it into the work environment.

While the creators of this metaphor do not explicitly reference the notion of a psychological instrument, we can observe that this cognitive aid exhibits all the characteristics of a genuine operative language for interpreting a procedural sequence within the environment. Beyond merely being a cognitive aid displayed on a specific medium, such as a poster on the wall, a notebook carried by caregivers or an image on a screen in the emergency room, the authors have extended this concept through various external tools for cognition (such as the emergency cart and signage) as well as internal ones (like the language logic for communication within the team). These tools facilitate the interchange between the cognition embedded in the work environment and that within the minds of the caregivers operating in that environment. Developing a cognitive aid in line with this usage logic of a psychological instrument, or essentially using a cognitive gateway, aims for a more structured thought process among its users.

2.2.2. *The structuring effect of psychological instruments*

Cognitive aids, classified as psychological instruments, facilitate the execution of a process of thought structuring. This structuring process involves the cognitive system, comprising the individual and their surrounding environment, learning, evolving and developing through their interactions.

More specifically, *in a first step, the individual externalizes their cognition by delegating it to an external psychological instrument*. Such an instrument serves as an alternative path for the natural flow of thought. This path is rooted in the environment through a device that provides a different way of reasoning, of processing information than the one typically used, such as the metaphor of the vortex for emergency oxygenation. Then, *in a second step, the use of external resources retroactively improves structuring, the functioning of internal cognition* (sharing an operative language facilitates a shared awareness of the situation, structures communications within the team around key terms). This is the step of internalization. Therefore, psychological instruments enable a back and forth between internal and external cognition. However, when the traveler makes their return journey, they are no longer the same, they have evolved. They have learned.

They have inherited modes of information processing provided through their journey.

A comprehensive illustration of this externalization/internalization process is the transition through writing. Writing serves as a psychological instrument itself, rooted in a broader psychological instrument, namely oral expression. To grasp this fundamental aspect of cognitive aids, we must delve into psychological instruments with a broader scope, those enabling both oral and written expression.

2.2.2.1. *Oral expression*

With the acquisition of language, a child gains a means of organizing and controlling their initially chaotic and unorganized thoughts. The child's world, initially composed of fleeting perceptual images, continually expands, enabling not only present but also past and future thinking, as well as the exploration of imaginary realms (Piaget 1937). Moreover, as language proficiency develops, the child significantly enhances their ability to communicate precisely with others, surpassing the limited expressive capacity provided by early life's basic behavioral responses such as sounds, cries, gestures, looks and movements. Communication transcends the immediacy of reactive sensations.

In certain circumstances among adults, oral expression can blatantly demonstrate its power as a psychological instrument serving thought. This is evident when a person has experienced a traumatic event. The traumatized individual may be unable to articulate what they saw, heard or felt. Oral expression then becomes the tool used by psychological support teams to help the victim mentally organize their experiences into a coherent sequence of events, fostering cognitive control gradually. When the victim verbally describes their experiences to the rescuer, the primary objective is not to inform the rescuer but to enhance the internal organization and control of distressing events.

As a means of communication, oral expression also offers additional advantages. This psychological instrument is highly efficient, given its close cognitive alignment with individual thought processes. Inner thoughts are often encoded verbally in short-term memory, facilitating a seamless transition to oral expression. Oral communication can smoothly transition from internal cognition, remaining as subvocal expression audible only to the speaker, to vocalized expression conveying thoughts to others. This continuum between internal and external cognition is further evidenced by the flexibility of oral communication.

In situations in which medical emergencies are being addressed by a team, professional guidelines emphasize *the importance of clear communication within the team to structure, coordinate and synchronize the activities of team members. Additionally, self-verbalization is also recommended as it enhances message processing in short-term memory*. However, oral expression, like any tool, has its limitations. It conveys a message that quickly dissipates with the acoustic wave carrying it. As a sound wave, vocal messages compete with other waves in the ambient acoustic environment. The message may become inaudible or distorted due to the presence of background noise (alarms, equipment noise, ongoing conversations). Vocal messages are impermanent, and their retention depends on the mental effort exerted by both the speaker and, particularly, the listener to remember the message content. Oral communication requires both the sender and the receiver to share the same space-time for the sound wave to reach its target.

With telecommunication instruments such as the telephone, it is possible to overcome the constraint of "sharing the same space", as communicators can be at a distance from each other. However, the temporal constraint of the shared moment persists unless a new instrument is used: sound recording. To surpass the constraint of the shared moment, the receiver must exert the effort to memorize the message for later rebroadcast. However, as psychologist Bartlett (1932) demonstrated long ago, a message transmitted orally within a group of individuals inevitably undergoes content distortion, which can be significant.

In the realm of medical emergency management by a team, the efficacy of using oral expression as a work aid is occasionally scrutinized. The acoustic environment and the multitude of exchanges can potentially impede each individual's capacity to concentrate on their task and to mentally vocalize the actions required (Chapelain et al. 2015). To surmount these limitations inherent in oral expression, humans have devised another psychological instrument, one that operates silently: written expression.

2.2.2.2. *Written expression*

Written expression possesses two objective characteristics that result in highly significant consequences for human cognition: the transfer of information from the auditory domain to both the visual and auditory domains, as well as the materialization of information through a physical medium.

2.2.2.2.1. A transfer from auditory encoding to both visual and auditory domains

The introduction of visual perception through reading, as well as during writing, offers the opportunity for additional information processing operations on the message, operations that are challenging to execute based solely on a fleeting oral message. Visualizing the message enriches it by situating it in space (top/bottom, left/right) and providing it with various forms (fonts, graphics, etc.). The visual representation of the message fosters the development of new cognitive skills such as reading and writing, which in turn enhance modes of thought expression. Even if the message becomes visual, it remains auditory during reading and writing, albeit at a subvocal level. *This dual coding process, in turn, enriches oral expression based on written expression.*

For instance, rhetoric is an oral formulation that necessitates prior deep analysis of content, thus requiring a transition through writing. The operative language derived from the metaphor of the vortex to assist in the management of a medical emergency exemplifies oral expression structured from written materials. This applies more broadly to communication protocols used in the medical field.

By way of illustration, the protocol for transmitting information in a care service, called the 4Ps (*purpose*, *picture*, *plan*, *part*), has the following communication scheme (Hansten 2003):

– *Purpose*: why is the patient here? What are the priorities?

– *Picture*: how can we describe the current state of the patient? What short- and long-term outcomes are we aiming for?

– *Plan*: what has worked and what has not?

– *Part*: what can be done next in the patient's management?

Such a protocol can be formulated very quickly orally (the advantage of oral expression), whereas it is based on a highly structured schema (the advantage of writing, which proved necessary during its design to select the critical information to be communicated). Here is an example of a quick and simple oral message heard in the emergency room during transmission, which can be analyzed through the 4Ps method: "Mr. X, acute drunkenness, head trauma (*purpose*), normal scan (*picture*), kept in to sober up (*plan*), be monitored (*part*)".

2.2.2.2.2. Materialization of information by writing

A particular property of graphic design (writing, drawing) is that *written information inherits the degree of permanence of its medium*. This stability is immeasurable compared to the duration of a verbal exchange. It provides every written document at least the potential to serve as an external memory aid, supporting internal memory processes. Through its materialization, writing becomes an object in itself, entering the cycle of objects within the human environment, involving stages of production, dissemination, use, preservation and maintenance. A written document can be distributed and shared among a very large group (space) and over a long period (time). On a cognitive level, the ability to reread a message allows for reflection and deep thought on the text. Anthropologist Jack Goody (1919–2015) convincingly demonstrated that the use of formal logic in human societies required the use of writing as a prerequisite. *Without writing, it is very difficult to scrutinize a statement, reflect on its validity or analyze it in depth.* In the workplace, cognitive aids most often use a written medium, whether paper-based or digital.

2.2.2.2.3. The disadvantages of writing

Like oral expression, written expression brings with it its constraints. Compared to oral communication, written production constitutes a less direct representation of thought. It requires additional specific operations both in the writing and reading phases. Reading and writing are operations that can take time. For example, during a resuscitation simulation exercise, in which we provided a document intended to recall elements of the procedure on a large screen, we observed the participants' difficulty in finding a moment to glance at the information, while they had no hesitation in exchanging oral communication among themselves and calling a specialist on the phone to obtain their opinion.

On the contrary, comprehension can also be more problematic than during verbal exchanges. Generally, unless notes are taken live on a blackboard, a text is read in the surrounding context that differs from the one in which it was written, leading to potential ambiguous interpretations. Additionally, the comprehension phase requires the development of a mental representation of the message, which is inherently more sophisticated than merely listening to a vocal message. Studies on document ergonomics have demonstrated the challenges posed by interpreting written instructions (Ganier 2018).

However, as an object in its own right, writing involves concrete manipulations that are added to the other actions specific to the main activity of the operators (retrieving, taking the document, flipping through it, replacing it in the initial place), not to mention all the operations necessary to access a document on a terminal when the document is in digital format, or the requirement of an electrical power source to operate the medium. Such manipulations are absent from oral communication. The proliferation of written materials contributes to the phenomenon of bureaucratization that pervades the world of work; it adds "additional checkboxes", to borrow one of the criticisms regarding the introduction of the surgical field checklist.

Finally, the materialization of knowledge on physical media carries the risk of assuming that the mere stable presence of these media suffices. If the user of the written document merely archives the knowledge in their environment, they risk losing the associated knowledge and skills. This passive archiving may be due to a lack of interest or the belief that we can rely on potentially accessible stored knowledge. However, this passive archiving often stems from documents that are not ergonomic, meaning they are difficult to access, lack reliability or do not inspire confidence in their use, to quote Clark and Chalmers (1998). To use the analogy of a gateway as describing a cognitive aid, we do not place a gateway between two points without designing it to be usable and without the objective of using it. Only the effective use of a document, in reading or writing, contributes to the functioning of the cognitive system, enabling the structuring of an individual's thoughts within this system. For a cognitive system to function, it must be dynamic, meaning cognitive resources can flow, bidirectionally, between its "individual" and "environment" components.

A highly illustrative example of a cognitive aid facilitating dynamic exchanges between a practitioner's knowledge and their informational environment is the software application "DansMaBlouse" developed by Guillaume Rieul, an anesthesiologist-resuscitator.

2.2.3. *A gateway between internal and external cognition: "DansMaBlouse" app*

The quest for information among practitioners is assuming a progressively greater role in their profession. This involves navigating the variability of care while considering the best available practices, staying abreast of the ongoing evolution of treatments and addressing the increasingly numerous and detailed inquiries from patients who themselves have access to varying degrees of reliable information on the Internet.

However, this requirement for information retrieval is time-consuming, as it involves gathering from multiple and diverse sources of information, in continually increasing quantities (medical manuals, specialist opinions, scientific articles, online databases, search engines, etc.). To organize this scattered information, medical students and practitioners use various mediums. Through a questionnaire completed by 148 medical interns, Rieul (2019) demonstrates that the storage media used are as follows in descending order: a handwritten notebook (36%), a USB flash drive (34%), a smartphone (30%), a medium that varies depending on the circumstances (27%), a computer (26%), loose sheets of paper (22%) and personal memory (14%).

Therefore, both in terms of information content and the mediums used, a broad spectrum is available to practitioners, requiring them to engage in genuine research and document management activity. The aim was therefore to consolidate this content and these mediums into a single integrative tool. This is the objective assigned to the software application "DansMaBlouse" (Figure 2.4), which means "in my gown" in French. In regards to content, documents are divided between a private space managed entirely by the user (referred to as "my gown pocket") and a shared space, facilitating information exchange between users with similar areas of expertise or interests (referred to as "shared gown pockets"). In terms of physical support, the information stored on a server is accessible both via computer and smartphone, the latter being a device extensively used by practitioners in their professional daily routines.

Therefore, the "DansMaBlouse" application truly represents a compelling example of the concept of a cognitive gateway. It serves as an informational mechanism for delivering a range of information from multiple sources to one or more users. Essentially, this gateway automates the process of disseminating information and knowledge, a task that previously required manual effort from medical professionals or medical students. By the end of February 2023, the free application, spread solely by word of mouth, boasted no fewer than 32,460 users across mainland France and the overseas territories. This serves as empirical evidence of the significant interest in a tool that gateways the gap between the external informational environment and the user's cognition.

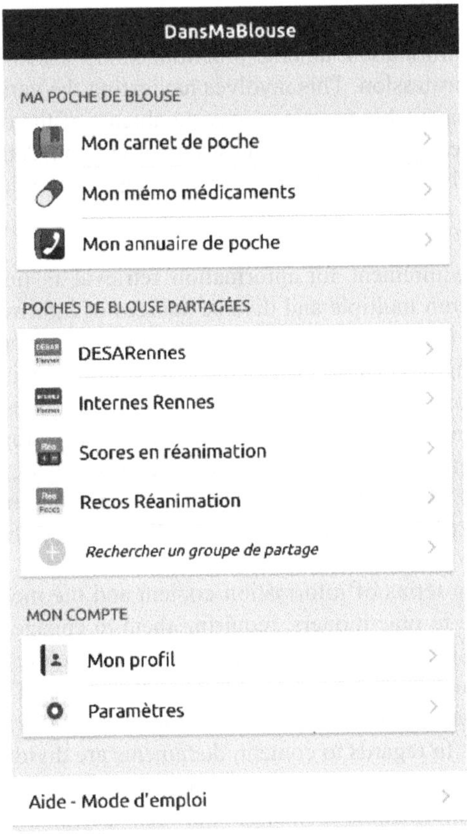

Figure 2.4. *Screenshot of the "DansMaBlouse" application.Reproduced with permission from Rieul (2019). For a color version of this figure, see www.iste.co.uk/morineau/cognitive.zip*

2.3. Conclusion

By opting to use a psychological instrument, thought is externalized and becomes reliant on a device. The inherent flow of thought then adopts the attributes of the employed instrument, including its structuring and the contributions made by its designers prior to use. This altered trajectory of thought represents a form of taming from its prior "wild" state (Goody 1979). However, for a cognitive aid to evolve into a genuine psychological instrument, it must possess a structuring capacity, effectively serving as a cognitive gateway to facilitate this new pathway of information and knowledge.

Concerns surrounding the automation of specific cognitive processing stages via cognitive aids could diminish if these aids facilitate both the externalization and internalization of knowledge in an ergonomic manner. In essence, the goal is for knowledge to depart from the brain only to return after traversing the environment, facilitated by a cognitive gateway. However, to be more precise, what are its points of departure, destination and return?

3

Routing Analytical Thinking to Support Intuition

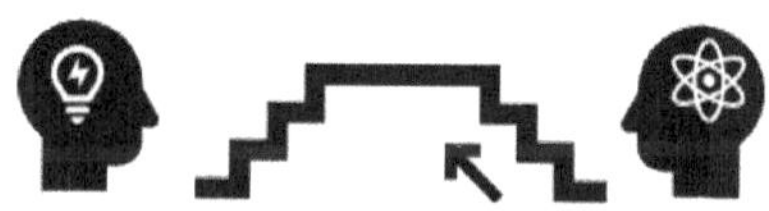

Figure 3.1. *Resources of analytical thinking (system 2) are brought to intuitive thinking (system 1)*

Conventionally, cognitive aid is primarily considered a "countermeasure" device put in place to avoid the occurrence of an error. A central issue in fields where cognitive aids, most often in the form of checklists, have spread (such as aeronautics, navigation, medicine, nuclear, etc.) is that of risk management. Human error is not tolerable when flying a plane or commanding a ship with hundreds of passengers on board, or when caring for fragile individuals in need of treatment. In the medical field, studies show that up to 75% of errors in general medicine originate from cognitive factors, affecting all stages of the diagnostic process, including information gathering, inference linking, contextual formulation, processing and verification. Error analysis in an American hospital setting suggests that at least 13% of diagnostic errors are related to the interpretation of test results and that 79% of errors occur during patient consultations. The risks are heightened as it appears that practitioners are not aware of the weaknesses in their reasoning. It has been shown that physicians who describe themselves as excellent decision-makers, attentive and unbiased, obtained low scores on a series of tests on medical cognitive biases (O'Sullivan et al. 2018).

The problem with the approach conventionally implemented in error analysis is that it tends to focus solely on the individual who has produced or is likely to produce an error. This approach often characterizes errors as "human", which is redundant, as ultimately a human will always be at the root of the causal chain leading to the error. This perspective leads to finding the nature of the failure "in the head" of an individual, whereas, as seen, every cognitive system inherently consists of both an individual and an environment. Psychologist James Reason, a prominent expert in error, summarizes the two major approaches to human error in this regard. The first approach, centered on the "individual", has long been dominant in organizations, particularly in the medical field. This approach views error as the violation of a procedure by an individual due to faulty or risky cognitive processes: forgetfulness, inattention, loss of motivation, negligence, recklessness. Cognitive aid is understood in this approach as a means of compensating for human reasoning weaknesses.

The second, more recent approach aims to consider error as a phenomenon emerging from the operation of a system that includes both individuals and their environment. Here, we encounter the notion of a cognitive system (Clark and Chalmers 1998). *While the individual-centered approach identifies the operator as the cause of the error, the system-oriented approach regards the production of an error as the consequence of malfunctions within the system.* When an accident or incident occurs, it represents the submerged part of the iceberg – a manifestation of latent failures that could have emerged at another time, in another form, perhaps even with different operators involved (Rasmussen 1990). The paradigm of error management is shifting: it is not solely about suppression but rather about avoiding, trapping and minimizing error and its consequences (Loyd et al. 2004).

However, the issue in studying cognitive aids is that one cannot inquire into their functions without delving into the intrapsychic mechanisms of information processing, which means focusing on the individual. Designing an appropriate cognitive aid involves devising a device tailored to how its future users reason, memorize and mentally represent the work situation and the task to be accomplished. While affirming that the relevant unit for understanding activity is the "individual–environment system", we must be able to focus the analysis on the "individual" component at a given moment. The challenge is therefore significant: How do we approach individual cognitive processes without falling into the trap of the individual-centered approach to characterizing error? To do this, we will attempt to zoom in on internal cognitive processes and their potential failures while keeping in mind the broader notion of the cognitive system. Very quickly, we will see the need to consider external cognition inserted into the environment to understand error and its regulation. The systemic approach will allow us to reintroduce cognitive aid as a gateway, not only between internal and external cognitions but also between different forms of internal cognitions, while taking a detour through the environment. Specifically, we will see that it is possible to establish gateways to route cognitive resources from analytical thinking to intuitive thinking.

Cognitive psychologists have long highlighted the sometimes surprising weaknesses that reasoning can exhibit during judgments or decision-making. Today, numerous studies on human factors, particularly in the medical field, with the authors often being physicians or nurses, demonstrate an appropriation of key concepts from the psychology of reasoning, such as cognitive biases or heuristics, to consider the flaws in reasoning in the realm of medical or paramedical decision-making. In particular, the theory of the dual cognitive system holds a central place in these studies. This theory distinguishes in humans, on the one hand, an intuitive system based on the automatic activation of information processing schemas, which is particularly susceptible to failures; and, on the other hand, an analytical system relying on conscious reasoning, adhering to the criteria of rational thought, where logical coherence is a guarantee of performance.

This dissociation between two cognitive systems was established long ago, originally suggested by the philosophers of ancient Greece (Croskerry 2009). In the Middle Ages, the philosopher William of Ockham made a clear distinction between abstract thinking and intuitive thinking. As a precursor, he demonstrated that the same object, whether concrete or abstract, could be understood by both modes of thought, while emphasizing that intuitive thinking, dealing with evidence, inherently prevailed over abstract thinking, which required a longer period of intellection (Piché 2005). Through experimental psychology, particularly the work of Tversky and Kahneman in the 1970s (Tversky and Kahneman 1974), this distinction has been empirically validated. One of the primary conclusions drawn from this experimental research is the identification of the vulnerability of intuitive thinking compared to analytical thinking.

3.1. Intuitive thinking: vulnerable thinking

Often, it is difficult to define what intuition is. However, if we refer to the theory of the dual cognitive system, this mysterious notion becomes clearer. Intuitive thinking (also called "system 1" or "type 1 process", as it is considered an archaic mode of thinking) consists of automated and rapid information processing mechanisms. Their implementation occurs unconsciously, with only the result provided by information processing typically reaching consciousness. The model that best illustrates the functioning of intuitive thinking is likely that of a semantic network composed of a set of nodes representing units of knowledge linked by connections symbolizing the relationships between these knowledge units. We can visualize this as a neural network. This model serves as the basis for research in artificial intelligence in the so-called "connectionist" approach. Through this model, two essential mechanisms help in understanding numerous psychological phenomena associated with intuitive thinking: network activation upon input (priming) and the strengthening of connections within the network (creation of knowledge schemas).

3.1.1. *Activation of the knowledge network: priming*

In intuitive thinking, the perception of information can initiate a network of knowledge. This activation propagates throughout a portion of the network, thereby activating certain units of knowledge already present. In his seminal book *Thinking, Fast and Slow*, Kahneman (2011) illustrates this priming phenomenon through an experiment in which subjects are presented either with the word "EAT" or "WASH". Following this exposure, they are asked to complete the missing letter in the word "SO_P". Participants who previously saw or heard the word "eat" predominantly perceive the word as "SOUP". Those who previously encoded the word "wash" see it as "SOAP". Therefore, the interpretation of new information occurs automatically based on previously received information (the initial activation of the network constituting the priming). They unconsciously serve as context, providing meaning. This automatic mode of triggering information processing allows for very rapid processing and hence the production of a direct adaptive response to a situation.

3.1.2. *Reinforcement of certain connections*

Within a network, certain connections between different nodes can strengthen due to the frequency of their activation. These reinforced connections lead to the development of knowledge schemas. Through the reinforcement of their links, these knowledge structures become organized sets through which the activation flow from priming diffuses automatically, without the effort of connecting knowledge. These schemas, sometimes also referred to as "scripts" (Abelson 1981), account for typical situations experienced by individuals. For example, the script "going to a restaurant" is developed in memory as the individual frequents this place. Once established, this script will be automatically activated upon arrival at a new restaurant. Within the script, the reinforced links between knowledge units create a set of expectations about what can be experienced in this situation: asking for a table, choosing dishes, being served, etc. As the individual visits a variety of restaurants, this schema may specialize into sub-schemas, each integrating the specifics of restaurants, thus refining expectations. By establishing a framework of expectations towards reality, schemas function as a set of a priori beliefs about how the world will present itself. A schema thus facilitates the coordination of inter-individual relationships in a given context through shared expectations. A common knowledge schema reduces explicit communications between individuals who share the same frame of expectations. The schema allows for anticipation of future events based on their likelihood of occurrence in light of the past. It speeds up information processing and reduces cognitive effort: there is no need to question the sequence of events to be experienced and the behaviors to adopt, either for ourselves or for others. One type of schema that particularly concerns decision-making is heuristics.

3.1.3. *Heuristics*

A heuristic is a schema that serves as *a shortcut in reasoning, facilitating rapid and a priori adapted judgments and decisions*. In the information processing chain proposed by the Rasmussen model (refer to Chapter 1), heuristics bypass certain steps in this chain. Unlike analytical reasoning, which involves strict adherence to the sequence of treatments, heuristics skip certain treatments. By recognizing simple cues in a situation, heuristics lead to an adaptive response. The most accurate way to describe a heuristic is to formulate it as a rule of the type "if such a condition, then such a decision/action" (Rasmussen 1986). This rule links a specific context (the condition) serving as a primer to an adaptive response. Like any knowledge schema, heuristics are based on the assumption that the environment is stable and has invariants.

An example of heuristics in the medical domain was articulated by a pediatrician during a debriefing session following simulator training in pediatric emergency procedures. The physician explained to colleagues that he relies on the beginning of the national anthem to recall the rhythm for initiating chest compressions during resuscitation. This strategy exemplifies heuristics for several reasons:

– it evolved from personal experience, extracting an invariant – the rhythm of compressions;

– it enables action initiation based on a cue from the perceived situation;

– it directly triggers a behavior deemed appropriate and effective;

– its theoretical content, explaining the link between the national anthem and compression rhythm, was not explicitly articulated or formalized. The heuristics emerged empirically from an association of ideas between musical rhythm (stored knowledge) and the rhythm of emergency maneuvers (lived experience);

– it can be formalized as a rule: "If beginning cardiac massage on a child, then internally hum the beginning of the national anthem and synchronize with it".

An interesting aspect of this example of cognitive aid is that it represents a heuristic informally discovered by a healthcare provider. However, a heuristic can ultimately lead to a shared and formalized knowledge schema. In the case of our example, it turns out that research, likely unknown to the pediatrician, has experimentally evaluated the potential contribution of different types of music to optimize the timing of resuscitation maneuvers (chest compressions and ventilations). For instance, in a study by Roehr et al. (2014), various musical pieces were compared in a simulated pediatric resuscitation exercise. Considering that the medical recommendations taken into account by the authors of the study at the time were a rate of 90 chest compressions and 30 ventilations per minute (current recommendations are 100–120 compressions per minute), Table 3.1 displays the average rates produced by participants under different experimental conditions: control condition "without music" or with five different types of music: four songs and one classical piece (Radetzky March). It turns out that the song *SOS* by the Swedish band ABBA gets closest to the recommended cadence (significant difference compared to the control condition). It is worth noting that the intuition of the doctor who independently chose the French national anthem was correct. Indeed, it has a rhythm of 123 beats per minute, which is close to the song *SOS*. Perhaps this slightly higher rhythm would even further approximate the medical recommendations.

Background music	Chest compressions/min	Ventilations/min
Control condition (without music)	80	28
***Stayin' Alive* (105 bpm)**	77	26
***Radetzky March* (110 bpm)**	80	27
***I Will Survive* (120 bpm)**	83	28
***Jingle Bells* (120 bpm)**	84	28
***SOS* (120 bpm)**	86	29

Table 3.1. *Observed rhythms during simulated resuscitation, with or without specific background music, according to Roehr et al. (2014)*

Heuristics are thus "strategies", discovered by an individual, potentially validated by a group of experts, enabling an efficient decision-making process in minimal time. However, experimental studies indicate that these strategies can also be misleading, producing errors in judgment, reasoning and decision-making. Psychological experiments reveal these errors, termed "cognitive biases". The significance of these biases sometimes leads to regarding the term "cognitive bias" as synonymous with "heuristics", as observed in numerous studies in social psychology.

3.1.4. *Cognitive biases*

Attuned to the revelation of human cognitive vulnerabilities, experimental psychologists, along with researchers in the human factors domain, have identified a plethora of cognitive biases. Enumerating them all would be tedious and uninteresting. To provide a rough estimate, physician and human factors specialist Pat Croskerry (2003) catalogues 22 cognitive biases in the medical field. Interestingly, it is possible to categorize them based on the general characteristics of a knowledge schema, distinguishing biases related to priming from those associated with highly interconnected knowledge nodes.

3.1.4.1. *Priming bias*

The observation that heuristics can be activated through mere priming is evident in the *anchoring effect*, which demonstrates that an initial judgment regarding an object influences subsequent judgments on that object or on an associated one. However, the contextual cue triggering the activation of a schema is not always relevant. For instance, a high price assigned to a consumer item primes the notion that the item is of high quality. This "price–quality" association has been established as a stable schema.

However, the prior activation of schemas can itself produce a priming effect. In the *availability bias*, the most recent and easily accessible knowledge schemas are preferred when considering a new situation. For instance, an emergency physician who has treated a heart attack may tend to prioritize this interpretation when faced with a second patient complaining of left arm pain.

A particular vulnerability of priming is its dependence on the superficial aspects of the situation. It is these superficial aspects that activate a specific schema. The *framing effect* represents this deceptive effect of appearances. In an experiment, Garcia-Retamero and Galesic (2010) presented participants with one of two scenarios: "Mr. Roe needs surgery. 9 out of 1,000 patients die following this surgery" or "Mr. Smythe needs surgery. 991 out of 1,000 patients survive this surgery." Participants were asked to assess the perceived risk of the surgical procedure on a four-point scale, ranging from 1 (no risk at all) to 4 (very risky). On average, participants judged that Mr. Roe had a higher risk of death following surgery than Mr. Smythe. The linguistic formulation of the problem gives the situation an appearance that leads to a biased interpretation.

Figure 3.2 depicts a graphical representation of the "Roe versus Smythe" problem. This graph, functioning as a simple psychological instrument, transforms into a genuine cognitive aid, helping to circumvent cognitive biases. Through its comprehensive display of survival and mortality probabilities, it mitigates the framing effect induced by linguistic formulation.

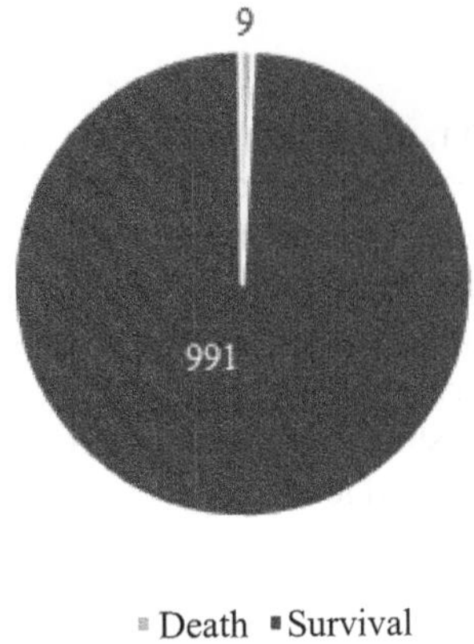

Figure 3.2. *Graphical representation of the risk of death following surgery*

3.1.4.2. *Bias linked to a reinforced network of knowledge*

The dominance of an activation network within a mental schema simplifies problem analysis by considering only the dimensions integrated into the schema. This reduces the possibility of exploring other interpretations or knowledge schemas. The internal coherence of the activated schema outweighs the external coherence, which would require analytical comparison between different alternatives to be validated.

A bias generated by this mode of operation is the *substitution bias*, which involves using simple reasoning where reasoning integrating multiple parameters would be necessary (Kahneman 2011). For example, at the onset of the Covid-19 pandemic, the massive influx of ICU patients led some decision-makers to focus solely on the availability of a sufficient number of ventilators or beds. However, these were only certain dimensions of the problem, because in addition to ventilators or beds, a set of other equipment, as well as a sufficient number of qualified personnel, were necessary. This bias is a substitution bias in the sense that a complex question is replaced by a more basic one (Landucci and Lamperti 2021).

The *confirmation bias* consists of seeking in the environment only the information that validates a previously posited interpretation. This bias represents the challenge of mentally deviating from an already activated and pre-structured thought pattern following a particular logic. This tunnel-like reasoning can be reinforced by *overconfidence bias*, which is the tendency to overestimate the validity of the intuitive reasoning that has just been activated.

On the contrary, intuitive thinking also relies on archaic adaptive response patterns that may influence how a situation is processed. This processing of basic information, found in all animals, is behavior based on affordances. Due to its rudimentary nature, this type of processing can lead to errors in assessing a situation.

3.1.5. *Affordance-based behavior*

Affordance is a term proposed by psychologist Gibson (1979). This term comes from the verb "to afford", which means "to provide". Gibson studied the mechanisms of perception and questioned this function from an ecological approach. His astonishment was about how simple animals, like a spider, could perceive objects in the environment essential for their adaptation and adjust accordingly, without having a sophisticated nervous system. An animal will be capable of perceiving in the environment areas usable as a medium to be traversed, surfaces serving as supports, or obstacles providing protection. Based on its own characteristics (size, volume, needs, etc.), a place will be perceived as an area in which to live or hide. Environmental objects are not objects with clearly defined and delimited usage modes. More than objects, an animal perceives, at the infraconceptual level where it operates when using affordances, properties offered by objects or areas available in the environment. This principle also applies to humans who can perceive a chair and consider it as an object to sit on, as well as a support to change a light bulb on the ceiling or as an object heavy enough to block a door. *In action, an animal thus does not see objects classified into predefined conceptual categories – linguistic categories specific to analytical reasoning – but a set of potential properties usable according to its current needs.* Perceiving the properties of the environment within the framework of a goal to be achieved triggers behaviors that integrate these properties. In the ecological approach, we find the logic of the "individual–environment" cognitive system.

However, like heuristics, affordance-based behaviors can be susceptible to perceptual appearances. Two types of errors can emerge: hidden affordances and false affordances (Gaver 1991). In the case of *hidden affordance*, the individual does not perceive certain properties in the environment that are nevertheless directly relevant to their adaptive needs. A typical example is a control button on an electronic device that is difficult to find. On a resuscitation room vacuum cleaner, the presence of both physical control buttons and touch control buttons can create confusion for the user. They may no longer know where to find the relevant controls. A hidden affordance for an animal would be the cat, a predator, camouflaged in the bushes next to the bird that does not see it.

In the case of *false affordance*, the organism is mistaken about the properties of an object or space. For humans, this is exemplified by the classic case of a door handle whose shape suggests pulling to open it, when in fact it should be pushed, or the scenario of the screen on the resuscitation room vacuum cleaner, which appears to feature a control button on the touch screen, though it does not (Coldewey et al. 2022). For our bird, it is the airspace that appears open for its movement, while a veranda window will obstruct it.

On a daily basis, humans engage in behaviors based on their habits (patterns, heuristics) and their perception of the properties of objects and spaces around them (affordances). However, *in the activities of healthcare providers, the complexity of certain clinical cases, which involve problem-solving, destabilizes routine patterns. The affordances typically used may no longer be relevant. Therefore, schemas and affordances need to be inhibited*. These destabilizations can lead to failures and errors. To address these risks, individuals must rely on cognitive resources beyond their intuitive thinking. These resources lie in their ability to base interpretations, decisions and actions on analytical thinking. According to cognitive psychologists, rational individuals must engage in analytical thinking to avoid cognitive biases and misleading affordances of intuitive thinking.

3.2. The power of analytical thinking

Analytical thinking (also known as "system 2" or "type 2 process") exhibits properties opposite to intuitive thinking. Analytical thinking is slow, processes information sequentially, and requires significant intellectual effort. Its control is conscious and relies on attentional resources distributed according to task demands: sustained attention on a task, resource allocation across multiple tasks and selection of information for processing. System 2 engages in analytical reasoning during decision-making by comparing and weighing different pieces of information. Pursuing comprehensiveness in considering cases and alternatives is essential for maintaining rationality. Analytical thinking involves calculations and data measurements. *Short-term memory*, also known as working memory, serves as the locus of analytical thinking (Baddeley 1992; Staal 2004).

While intuitive thinking manipulates the relationships between knowledge units implicitly or bypasses certain steps, analytical thinking is characterized by the explicit articulation of the sequence of information units involved in reasoning. In the context of analytical reasoning, the equivalent of connections between nodes in intuitive schemas corresponds to inferences. French psychologist Pierre Oléron (1915–1995), who studied human intelligence, defined inference as follows: "Inference consists of the passage from a given or initial assumption to an assumption that is accepted because of its connection with the former" (Oléron

1977, p. 57). This idea reflects the connections between knowledge units that constitute schemas in intuitive thinking. However, in the case of inferences, these connections are made explicit and constructed transiently during the course of reasoning. Oléron distinguished elementary or immediate inferences – which correspond to intuitive thinking (the network of connections between knowledge units) – from proper reasoning, which involves the development of a potentially large number of inferences that combine. Developing analytical reasoning is therefore cognitively costly.

> Short-term (or working) memory is composed of:
>
> – an attentional system that ensures the engagement of attentional resources on selected information (sustained, divided, selective attention);
>
> – an articulatory–phonological loop that allows the use of language as a mode of encoding vocal or subvocal information, as well as reading and writing;
>
> – a visuo-spatial system enabling the development of mental images that enrich the representation of a situation;
>
> – an episodic buffer serving to maintain short-term events that have just been experienced.

Box 3.1. *Components of short-term or working memory (Baddeley 1992)*

3.2.1. *Natural language and analytical thinking*

To form inferences, explicitly articulate and construct connections within a set of information, analytical thinking can initially rely on the capacity of language articulation. Indeed, verbal exchanges are based on the explicit expression of each individual's thoughts and, as seen with the psychological instrument notion, language also serves to clarify our own initially vague thoughts. As noted by Oléron, effective communication is considered to occur when the speaker's words are sufficiently explicit, avoiding any confusion or misunderstanding. However, natural language rarely achieves a level of reasoning articulation where the entire chain of inferences is clearly formulated. In everyday life, verbal exchanges are based on both an explicit aspect, the message conveyed by the speaker, and an implicit aspect, the cognitive context necessary for understanding this message.

In cognitive linguistics, the relevance theory proposed by Sperber and Wilson (1989) illustrates the interplay between the explicit and the implicit in communication. Upon receiving a message that is articulated orally or in writing, the receiver searches in their memory (internal cognition) or immediate environment (external cognition) for a cognitive context that allows them to interpret the message correctly. The authors refer to this as the "contextual effect". This pertinent context is implicit. For example, when Thomas tells Véronique, "I spoke to Sandrine on the phone yesterday. She's doing well", this statement refers to a context in which the person mentioned, Sandrine, is known to both interlocutors. Moreover, the exchange highlights the fact that this person is doing well, which may refer to a context in which this has not always been the case, indicating that she has experienced difficult events known to the interlocutors as well. Here, we have the sharing of implicit information stored in memory. However, language can also implicitly refer to the environmental context, here and now. For instance, when Thomas tells Véronique, "I prefer this one", the implicit aspect that allows the message to be understood is localized to where the object is pointed to by Thomas's finger.

This use of implicit information can lead to shortcuts in reasoning. Oléron provides an illustration: if two statements are presented to a sample of people, "The bird is in the cage. The cage is under the tree", a significant proportion of participants will believe they read: "The bird is under the tree". In doing so, they have unconsciously omitted two inferences: one connecting the bird to the cage and the other connecting the cage to the tree. An inferential shortcut is made, which is a process similar to that involved in the development of heuristics.

The implicit nature of language makes it prone to misunderstandings and even misinterpretations if the shared cognitive context is not accurately established between the interlocutors or between the writer and the reader of a text. While analytical thinking, which aims to clarify chains of reasoning, helps to avoid errors, the ideal would be to go beyond natural language and produce a comprehensive explanation of all the steps in the reasoning chain. This objective is the one pursued by formal logic.

3.3. Formal logic to elucidate reasoning

In a remarkably clear manner, Gottlob Frege (1848–1925), a renowned logician, mathematician and philosopher, formulated the following objective as he studied formal logic: "To prevent anything intuitive from creeping in unnoticed, every effort should be made to ensure that the chain of inferences contains no gaps" (Begriffsschrift 1979; Rivenc 1989). In other words, all inferential links connecting the various pieces of information embedded within the chain of reasoning should be explicit. Logic helps to avoid the ambiguity often found in natural language, as well as the polysemy of statements stemming from implicit meanings. To achieve this goal, a method of reasoning is required that starts from premises and leads to a conclusion via a sequence of explicit inferences, such as syllogism. Mathematics is closely tied to formal logic. It can be viewed as the quantitative counterpart to the qualitative statements expressed in logic. The calculations made possible by mathematics represent a thorough explanation of the properties and laws of the entities hidden behind numbers. Needless to say that logical–mathematical propositions can be particularly demanding in cognitive effort. Moreover, it is noteworthy that algebraic representations pertain to a linguistic formulation, like that facilitated by the articulo-phonological loop, while geometric representations relate to the visuo-spatial system, i.e. two components of short-term memory. Although geometric figures may appear intuitive due to their graphical nature, this is a deceptive impression; they constitute true abstractions.

3.3.1. *Navigating towards analytical thinking without assistance*

Psychologists, following Kahneman's research, have investigated the two modes of thinking (system 1 and system 2) in laboratory settings, often with students as participants. They have demonstrated that errors in problem-solving arise from the failure to engage in analytical reasoning, which could lead to finding the correct solution. Apart from the lack of intellectual skills required for analytical thinking, several factors related to information processing hinder access to analytical thinking:

– difficulty in inhibiting intuitive responses;

– high cognitive cost of attentional effort;

– inability to explicate certain knowledge schemas.

3.3.1.1. *Difficulty in inhibiting an intuitive response*

A preliminary process for the activation of analytical thinking is inhibition or, in other words, the blocking of intuitive thinking. Inhibition allows for cognitive control (Norman and Shallice 1980; Houdé 1995). This preliminary inhibition is challenging because schemas, heuristics and affordances can be activated very quickly, without delay, as soon as they are primed, while the activation of analytical reasoning takes longer. As William of Ockham foresaw, at the outset of information processing, intuitive thinking prevails over analytical thinking. Once a schema has been introduced, it continues to unfold without offering the opportunity to understand the situation in a different way to that characterized by the schema. This is indicated by some cognitive biases, such as confirmation bias.

The cognitive competition between intuition and analysis to interpret a situation is experimentally observable through a simple task, known as the "Stroop effect", named after the author of this task (Scarpina and Tagini 2017). In this neuropsychological test, participants are presented with a series of colored words. The peculiarity of this list is that the words are in a different color to the one they express (e.g. the word "red" is written in blue). However, participants are instructed to name the colors of the words rather than read the words, as quickly as possible.

This task leads to errors as participants tend to read the written word rather than name its color. In this task, the automatic reading schema that typically initiates when processing a word presented in writing competes with naming the colors of the font, which is a non-automated process. To name the color, we must first inhibit the reading process, which, with the speed instruction given to participants, tends to dominate. Significant attentional control effort is required to achieve this inhibition.

In the field of healthcare, as in any work scenario, there are situations in which a specific effort to inhibit routine patterns is necessary in order to enable a reasoned and appropriate response.

One example of a challenge related to the inhibition process concerns the resuscitation of a newborn. This task in particular demands rapidly providing adequate oxygenation to the infant. However, this strategy differs from adult resuscitation, which requires a particular focus on performing chest compressions to reactivate the cardiorespiratory system. During simulator exercises, healthcare providers report the temptation to immediately perform chest compressions on the newborn, as resuscitating adults is a more common scenario in emergency medicine than newborn resuscitation. This operational mode is based on a well-integrated script.

This inhibition mechanism is also a significant issue in managing crisis situations, particularly during a massive influx of victims following a disaster. At the appropriate moment, teams must inhibit their usual mode of operation to transition to a different mode, known as "degraded" mode. Therefore, the strategy known as damage control requires that doctors do not delve deeply into the care of each victim. Instead, they must quickly diagnose all victims to prioritize interventions based on their level of urgency. However, this strategy contradicts the usual approach of doctors, who typically focus on thorough care for the first patient they examine.

3.3.1.2. *Attentional effort and mental workload*

Inhibiting a knowledge schema that carries cognitive biases will be facilitated by an attentional effort. This implies that:

> [clinicians] must be informed and recognise the need for constant vigilance and surveillance of their thinking to mitigate diagnostic and other clinical errors. There is an ongoing imperative to self-monitor for bias and especially to be mindful of faulty decision making at vulnerable times, and for the risk of excessive reliance on intuitive

judgements when further reflection is required (Croskerry et al. 2013, p. 70).

However, such self-supervision involves a significant mental load, in addition to the burden associated with processing multiple demands in the work environment. In the context of training nursing students for their internship periods and subsequent professional practice, they are required to consistently engage in analytical thinking. This analytical thinking corresponds to what is termed "clinical judgment". Clinical judgment involves a rigorous reasoning process comprising several steps:

– Identifying patient symptoms that highlight deviations from expectations, rather than relying on recognizing typical situations as dictated by intuition. This identification process involves searching for additional potential information to avoid tunnel vision information processing typical of knowledge schemas.

– Interpreting based on data prioritization. This interpretation also involves searching for rational explanations if the initial interpretation was made intuitively. This requires inhibiting interpretations that are not sufficiently explicit.

– Responding by developing a planned and sufficiently explicit intervention. This clarity in intervention aims to facilitate clear communication with the patient and their family.

– Reflecting retrospectively on the reasoning process to evaluate its quality against expectations and draw lessons from it.

Such an endeavor becomes even more demanding as students are also required to engage in reasoning about their reasoning. In fact, clinical judgment should ideally be the subject of a process of self-reflection to improve judgment. This reflection on reflection, known as "critical thinking", falls within the domain of what is termed metacognition (Paul and Heaslip 1995; Maudsley and Strivens 2000; Simpson and Courtney 2002). It aims to enable students to increase their level of awareness in correctly implementing analytical reasoning.

Table 3.2 presents examples of questions regarding critical thinking. In this context, the following is noteworthy: "In the case of intuition, what type of data could offer evidence that supports your intuition?", a question aimed at providing analytical arguments to an interpretation based on intuition.

Within the range of ways to strengthen our own attentional control, so-called *debiasing or forcing strategies* are proposed to help the activation of analytical reasoning (O'Sullivan et al. 2018). These strategies aim to offer healthcare providers the following.

Tanner model phase	Clinical judgment category	Example questions
Identify	Sustained observation	What did you notice first about the patient?
	Recognizing deviations from expectations	What was different from your expectations? Have you seen this in a patient before?
	Seeking additional information	What other information would be useful? How can you obtain this information?
Interpret	Data prioritization	How did you prioritize the patient's information? What is now most important for this patient?
	Making sense of data	On what did you base your choice of intervention? In the case of intuition, what type of data could provide evidence that supports your intuition?
Respond	Calm and confidence	What was your approach with the patient? Did you feel comfortable?
	Clear communication	How do you think you can gain the patient's trust? What did you tell the patient, their family?
	Well-planned/flexible intervention	What factors (including patient feedback) influenced the care plan?
Reflect	Considering judgment quality	Did you perform skillfully compared to nursing standards?
	Assessment/self-analysis	What went well? What was not as evident as expected? Why?
	Commitment to improvement	What would you have done differently if given the opportunity?

Table 3.2. *Examples of questions to stimulate critical thinking among nursing students, based on Lasater (2011)*

– Education on cognitive biases and how to counteract them, as well as instruction on how to deal with statistics that frequently carry cognitive biases.

– An interesting strategy is to encourage operators to impose a slowing down of their decision-making processes, thereby increasing the chances of activating analytical reasoning.

– As part of the recommendations contained in the critical thinking method, another strategy is to systematically self-evaluate our own decisions by assigning them a confidence score.

During the course of study in health sciences, it is crucial to teach both educators and students the mechanisms of clinical reasoning and to cultivate metacognitive strategies in them. Once they become professionals, it is observed that half of the errors result from reasoning issues (Pelaccia et al. 2011), and every year, 5–15% of students with reasoning difficulties enter the healthcare market (Audétat 2012). Thierry Pelaccia (2016b) considers teaching the mechanisms of clinical reasoning to be a public health priority. Throughout the training program, the exercise to deploy reasoning about reasoning is an opportune moment. However, as students transition into professionals, metacognitive strategies add to the short-term memory workload, which already includes ongoing tasks that require attention. For instance, it is challenging to pose all the questions presented in Table 3.2 after each daily decision. This difficulty is compounded by the fact that some knowledge manipulated by intuition is not readily accessible to consciousness and thus falls outside the realm of metacognitive control.

3.3.1.3. *Inability to articulate certain knowledge schemas*

A limitation in the ability to engage in analytical thinking resides in the unconscious nature of the content of activated schemas. This refers to tacit knowledge or implicit learning. Throughout various adaptations individuals must undergo, they evolve and learn unconsciously. A typical context for implicit learning is the acquisition of a second language. While there are teachings and manuals that provide vocabulary, grammar and semantics based on predominantly explicit knowledge, true mastery of a language often requires immersion in a country for several months or regularly watching television in the language.

The experimental demonstration of the existence of implicit learning was conducted in a remarkable way by Reber (1989). One of his flagship experiments was as follows: an imaginary formal grammar describing the grammatical rules governing sequences of uppercase letters was devised in advance by the experimenters. This grammar made it possible to determine whether any sequence of letters was grammatically correct or incorrect according to arbitrarily established rules (e.g. the sequence ABXT would be correct, but AXTB would not). Once this grammar was constructed and hidden from the participants, a series of letter sequences was presented to them. They were instructed to memorize them, knowing that they were told that all these sequences were correct according to a certain grammar. After this phase, participants had to intuitively judge whether new sequences of letters, not belonging to the previously seen sample, were correct or not. The results indicate that, on average, participants succeed in judging whether a sequence is correct or not, even though they had never had access to the grammar governing it. At the end of the exercise, when participants were asked to describe what they thought the grammar was governing the sequences they evaluated, they were unable to explain it, even though they demonstrated mastery in practice (Cleeremans et al. 1998).

In the professional domain, an example of implicit learning pertains to the activity of submariners specializing in acoustics. These operators, known as the "golden ears", are tasked with identifying the acoustic signature of vessels circulating around the submarine during its immersion. A team of ergonomists responsible for developing an assistance system for these operators had the mission of asking these specialists to describe the sound signature specific to different types of vessels. However, they were unable to explain their process. Similarly, explaining how to ride a bike to a young child is challenging. The best solution is to put them on the bike…

On the contrary, social psychology has demonstrated that access to the consciousness of implicit reasoning can be impeded by psychological barriers, particularly when individuals exhibit behavior contrary to their ideas or values. The *cognitive dissonance* between behavior and values leads individuals to offer false explanations for their actions, aiming to avoid challenging their values or beliefs. This extensively studied phenomenon in social psychology is referred to as the *cognitive rationalization bias* (Joulé and Beauvois 2002).

These difficulties, sometimes leading to an impossibility, along with the cognitive cost associated with transitioning to analytical thinking, demonstrate the challenge for an isolated individual, caught up in their own reasoning, to avoid the cognitive biases of intuitive thinking. In such an individual-centered approach to cognition, solutions to overcome these obstacles are difficult to propose. There is a risk of quickly falling into the bias of interpreting the situation in terms of insufficient skills or a lack of attentional effort. This leads to attributing the cause of poor performance solely to the individual. However, framing the problem in this way is flawed. It either focuses on the mental capabilities or the motivation of the individual. Yet, if we consider the cognitive system as a whole, solutions exist within the "environment" component. These solutions are cognitive aids that will channel analytical resources to support intuitive thinking.

3.3.2. *Routing analytical resources through cognitive aid*

Müller-Lyer's perceptual illusion serves as a straightforward example to illustrate the role of an external resource in providing analytical reasoning.

3.3.2.1. *An example of analytical input: Müller-Lyer illusion*

In the Müller-Lyer illusion, when observing the two horizontal lines, for the majority of observers, it appears that the top line is longer than the bottom line (Figure 3.3). This illusion is explained by the priming of a perceptual schema. This schema implicitly uses the oblique lines on the sides as cues for judging the length of each line. We could characterize these cues as affordances that automatically guide perceptual judgment. However, these cues are false affordances, since both lines are actually of the same length. As Kahneman (2011) notes, it is sufficient to use a ruler to verify that the two lines are of equal length. For the author, the ruler provides an objective measurement of the length of the lines. This measurement represents the implementation of analytical thinking.

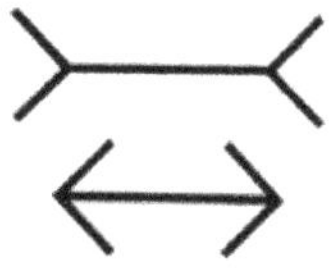

Figure 3.3. *Müller-Lyer's perceptual illusion*

However, in our opinion, Kahneman simplified the description of this moment of transition. Indeed, he fails to point out that, without the graduated ruler, the transition to an analytical perception of the figure could not have been made. In other words, *the rationality of the measurement is physically carried by the instrument.*

If we detail this use of the graduated ruler as a cognitive aid, different steps can be specified.

– *Stopping information processing, inhibition*: initially, to use the graduated ruler, we must inhibit the initial impression given by the intuitive perception of the illusion, to doubt it and question it.

– *Seeking external resources, externalization*: this blocking process involves exploring the environment to find a way to accurately assess the length of the lines. The individual chooses to rely on an external instrument present in their surrounding environment, a resource that is accessible to them.

– *Routing resources inward, internalization:* the actual measurement of the line lengths constitutes the routing of the cognitive resource provided by the graduated ruler to the internal cognition of its user (Figure 3.4). The ruler is considered a *reliable* tool in which we can *trust* to obtain an accurate measurement of the line.

It is worth noting that if a graduated ruler had not been available in the immediate environment, another cognitive aid could have been used to access the analytical resources: a strip of paper cut out, or even a simple spacing of the fingers – any device capable of serving as a material invariant for calculating the lengths of the figure. The cut-out strip of paper or the spacing of the fingers would constitute cognitive aids created by the user, while the graduated ruler is a pre-designed instrument for measuring length. In one case, the user employs an aid provided in their environment, while in the other, they design their own cognitive aid to address an ad hoc problem. It is also noteworthy that using the fingers to measure distance involves tapping into bodily cues. This illustrates the continuum between the external and internal environments within a cognitive system. The body serves as the interface between these two components.

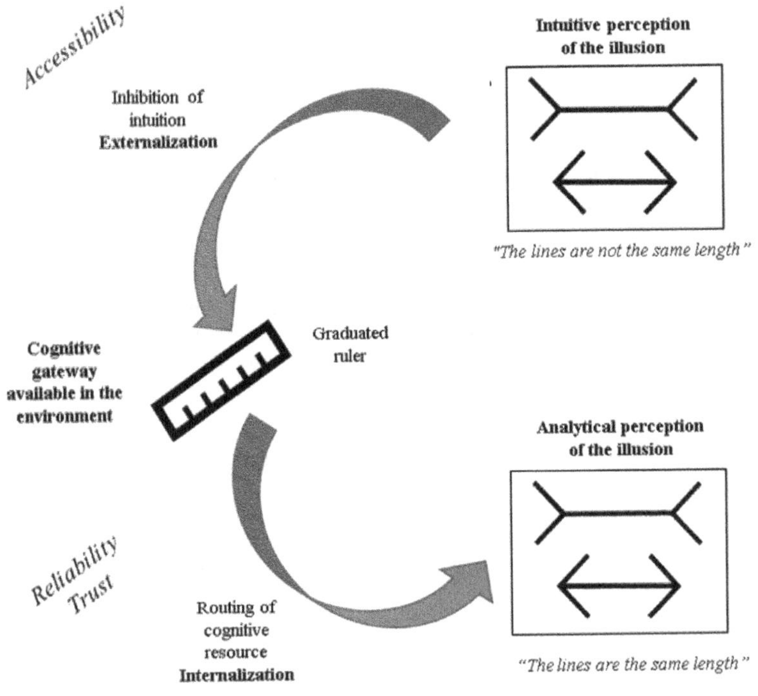

Figure 3.4. *Transition from intuitive to analytical perception with the assistance of a graduated ruler*

Kahneman's underestimation of the role played by the graduated ruler as a material tool for analytical thinking is indicative of an exclusively individual-centered approach to cognition. In general, this type of laboratory experiment focuses on observing the cognitive pitfalls that naive participants (students) can fall into when immersed in an empty and artificial environment (the laboratory). A new experiment that would provide a ruler to the participants to show its usefulness in dispelling the optical illusion would have no scientific interest; its result would be trivial. In a sense, the same type of result is obtained when measuring the percentage of expected actions performed by a team of healthcare professionals who have a checklist displaying the expected actions in question. All other things being equal, it "suffices" to follow the items on the checklist to achieve the expected result or a result close to it (a high percentage of checklist compliance). In terms of academic problem-solving situations, this falls into the realm of the trivial.

In natural problem-solving contexts, this scenario becomes non-trivial. Using an instrument to reach a solution reflects an essential human skill: instrumental competence. In real-world settings, especially in work contexts, individuals are surrounded by psychological instruments. These instruments play a pivotal role in mitigating the cognitive biases inherent in intuitive thinking by providing direct access to analytical resources within the surrounding environment. The effectiveness of these instruments in facilitating activity varies depending on their perceived reliability and accessibility in context.

The significance of this cognition integrated into the environment has already been highlighted through concepts such as "situated cognition" (Suchman 1987) or "distributed cognition" (Hutchins 1995). However, the role of cognitive gateways provided by certain components of this environment has not, to our knowledge, been sufficiently emphasized and fully considered as a conceptual framework for understanding and designing cognitive aids.

3.3.2.2. *Instruments for knowledge development*

Enabling access to analytical thinking through a cognitive gateway to mitigate the biases of intuitive thinking requires further explanation of information. Consider a simple list comprising a series of items. *The list serves as an initial form of clarification*, facilitating the structuring and organization of thought (Goody 1979). It provides:

– *storage on a permanent medium*: paper materializes the information that can be physically manipulated and preserved over a long period;

– *decomposition of the continuous flow of oral expression into distinct units*: each item is isolated, separated from others, through its position in the list. Each item synthesizes information. They are often keywords that constitute an abstraction of information;

– *rigor, comprehensiveness*: a list has a beginning and an end, as well as an assumed completeness;

– *arrangement of information*: the presentation order of items can itself provide additional information. A specific criterion can determine this order: the degree of importance, the sequence to follow, alphabetical order for indexing, etc.;

– *possibilities for active processing*: the list can be read in different ways and can be annotated (crossing out items that have been dealt with). Typically, the checklist used in the workplace is a highly structured list.

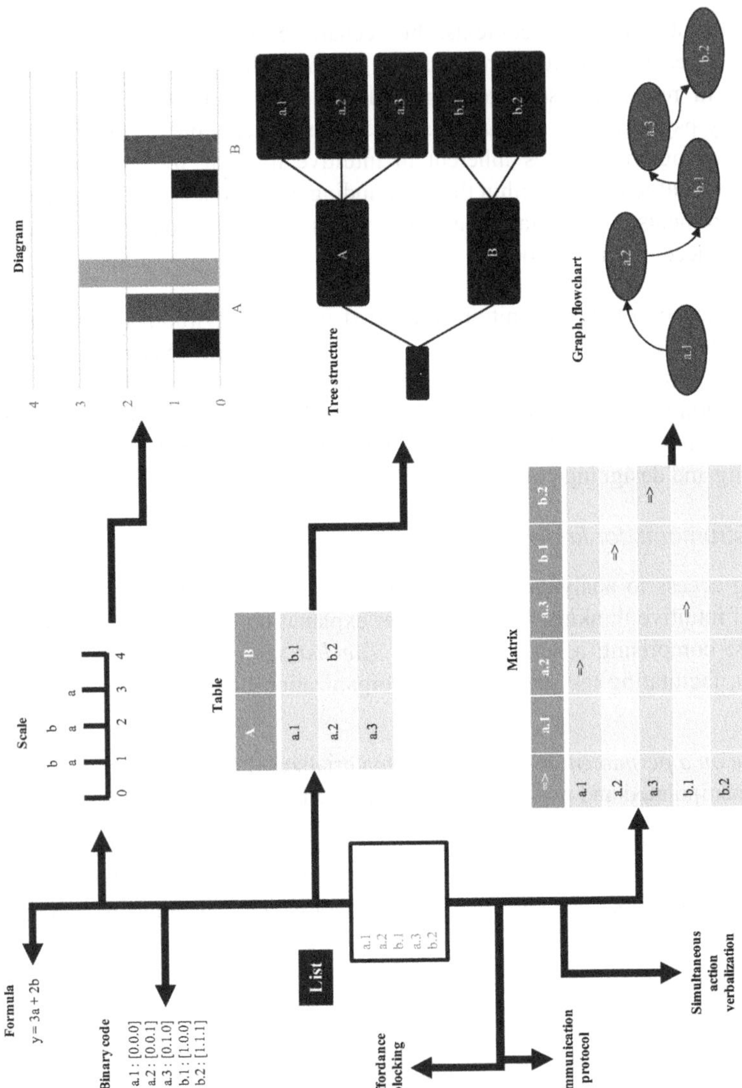

Figure 3.5. *Cognitive gateways facilitating access to analytical thinking from a simple list of items*

Beyond the simple list, numerous cognitive gateways can be conceived. They provide the option of highlighting certain properties of the information that the designer wishes to emphasize to assist users. Figure 3.5 presents a set of gateways that can be derived from a simple list. This enumeration is not exhaustive, but it demonstrates the variety of instruments that can be created to route analytical resources. Each type of instrument allows for the clarification of certain properties of the information contained in the list. In Figure 3.5, we find different representations that refresh the same series of items composing the initial list (the items denoted here as "a1, a2, b1, a3, b2").

– *The table*: this instrument adds additional order to the list. It materializes a classification, establishing relationships of belonging/exclusion by grouping the items into distinct sets. The table can be graphically represented in the form of a tree structure. Didactic materials frequently use this type of representation to describe a field of knowledge. Developed based on a temporal criterion, the table will bring forth other instruments such as the agenda or the calendar. These instruments allow for the planning of future events and the preservation of their trace along the timeline. Through them, time can be explicitly represented.

– *The matrix*: this is a double-entry table with the unique feature of intersecting multiple variables or a variable with itself. By intersecting the modalities of a variable with itself, it becomes possible to identify the relationships existing between these modalities within the cells of the matrix. For instance, if each column/row represents a state, it allows for exhaustive identification of the relationships between these states. Completeness is a key aspect of analytical thinking. Such analysis enables the generation of transition graphs between states, making clear the nature of relationships between different elements. These graphs may manifest as flowcharts or algorithms. The graph accentuates the sequential articulations within the information, such as causal relationships and logical implications.

– *The measurement scale*: it transcends the limitations of a table, which typically embodies a binary relationship of "belongs" or "does not belong" to a category. Instead, items are positioned along a scale, enabling their ordering and quantification, thus yielding synthetic measurement indicators such as total or average scores derived from the items listed. In the medical field, the Glasgow Coma Scale, used to assess a trauma victim's level of consciousness, exemplifies this cognitive aid for quantifying items originally of a qualitative nature (such as eye opening, verbal response and motor response). Once quantified, the data can be represented in various diagrammatic forms (e.g. histograms, curves), facilitating visualization and the discernment of specific properties that are otherwise difficult to perceive.

– *The equation*: in our example, we observe that the list comprises *3 items a + 2 items b*. An equation embodies a mathematical syntax enabling the multiplication of operations on information content by introducing constants, variables and facilitating reformulations and the identification of unknowns. Equations facilitate mathematical modeling, which, in turn, facilitates predictive analysis of phenomena, serving as high-level decision support.

– *Binary coding*: this constitutes a form of information mathematization grounded in Shannon's information theory. This theory enables the encoding of a message into binary units termed "bits", a familiar unit of measurement in computer science. The binary coding of "yes/no" checklists adheres to this logic of binary information quantization. Beyond checklists and closed-ended questions in a questionnaire, binary code facilitates computer modeling (one byte = 8 bits), thus enabling the design of highly complex cognitive aids such as digital terminals.

– *Verbalization concomitant with action*: reading a list aloud aids in its processing in short-term memory. By prompting operators to articulate their actions aloud, a shift occurs in short-term memory involving cognitive attentional control. In a simulation room experiment involving nursing students, the experimenter, stationed in the control room, communicated with participants via a walkie-talkie and earpiece. At specific intervals, the experimenter would inquire, "Tell me what you're doing right now". During one such inquiry, a student was administering a medication dosage. Requesting her to articulate her actions allowed her to recognize an error in the dosage (Chapelain et al. 2015). In emergency care practices, concurrent verbalization has become standard, particularly to ensure the verification of medication preparations.

– *Communication protocols*: they serve as a framework for organizing exchanges to systematically deliver a set of key information. Designing a communication protocol requires prior analytical reflection on the nature of the information to be transmitted. In the United States, the frequency of transmissions in a teaching hospital is estimated at 4,000 per day, highlighting the significant nature of this activity. A study by the Joint Commission across 10 hospitals indicates that transmission receivers estimate the proportion of unsuccessful transmissions at 37%. Senders rate this proportion at 21%. Reasons include delays in message reception, lack of attention during exchanges and insufficient information obtained about the patient in question. Streamlining verbal exchanges through communication protocols helps to mitigate these risks.

– *Affordance blocking*: we have seen that using an external cognitive aid to counter an uncertain-value intuition requires inhibition, a blocking of intuition. One way to protect against affordances that automatically trigger behavior is to establish real or symbolic barriers, thereby facilitating analytical reasoning. By adhering to the sequence of items described in a list, the operator can avoid being drawn into the solicitations around them, which may disrupt their structured workflow. The "sterile cockpit" in aviation, where no disturbances should occur through verbal exchanges during certain critical phases of flight, is an example of affordance blocking: the pilot may be there to hear what others want to say, but it is necessary not to disturb them. Medication preparation areas displaying a "do not disturb" sign operate on the same principle. The presence of floor tapes in an emergency care room, delineating the space dedicated to each caregiver based on their role around the patient, is a form of blocking chaotic movements. In an experiment with this setup, it was shown that these delineations made healthcare providers feel more capable of multitasking and objectively reduced mutual disruptions (Morineau et al. 2017).

We are thus faced with a set of basic cognitive gateways capable of serving as frameworks for the development of aids to analytical thinking or, in other words, for the manipulation of properties that would remain hidden if they were left to intuitive thinking. These clarifications help to avoid cognitive biases, false affordances or hidden affordances. Today, data scientists are typically specialists in recoding data for in-depth analysis. Their task is to explain the properties of a dataset, presenting them from the most relevant angle to guide decision-making. They can thus be described as designers of aids for analytical decision-making.

3.4. Conclusion

By focusing on internal processes, cognitive psychology research inadvertently supports an individual-centered approach to understanding errors in the workplace. In this logic, access to analytical thinking that avoids cognitive biases can only be achieved through individual intellectual effort to inhibit basic reasoning patterns, exert significant attentional resources, deploy chains of logical inferences or develop metacognitive reasoning capable of evaluating the quality of our own inferences. These are cognitive tasks that are difficult to implement for an individual considered in isolation, lacking any external resources to assist them. Resources distributed in the environment are not included in the cognitive analysis of the situation.

To address this issue of cognitively costly information processing, it is necessary to move away from focusing solely on the individual and instead consider the relevant unit as the global cognitive system including its environment. Naturally, humans introduce pre-existing or on-the-spot created psychological instruments to support their reasoning: lists, rules, formulas, tables, concomitant verbalization, etc. These instruments represent an externalization and then an internalization of knowledge units. These knowledge units are carried by a gateway, which is often both material and symbolic (e.g. the ruler and its millimeter scale, the sheet of paper and its diagram, etc.). If the instrument is easily accessible, reliable and can be trusted to achieve the task's objective, then it will fully play the role of a cognitive gateway between vulnerable intuition and rigorous analysis.

However, if we are indeed discussing cognitive gateways, we should also observe pathways of cognitive resources in the opposite direction, i.e. coming from intuitive thinking and supporting analytical thinking. To consider such devices, we would first need to accept that, in some cases, it is intuition that is capable of supporting analytical thinking and that there are psychological instruments that facilitate this process. In other words, a small paradigmatic revolution in relation to the classical approach to cognition.

4

Routing Intuitive Thinking to Support Analysis

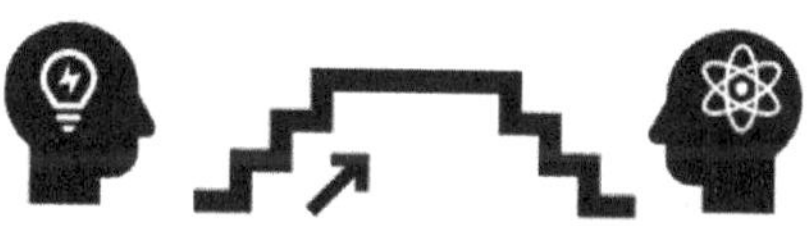

Figure 4.1. *Intuitive resources (system 1) that are brought to analytical thinking (system 2)*

Laboratory experiments on human reasoning during problem-solving have long propagated the notion of a standard of reasoning used as a benchmark to evaluate subjects' responses. This standard is formal logic, which represents the most sophisticated means of explicating statements. Formal logic serves as a yardstick to assess the quality of thought. The dual-system theory (intuitive/analytical thinking) has infiltrated this paradigm, positing analytical thinking as the optimal strategy to circumvent cognitive biases. Given that many psychology researchers are also educators, it became natural for them to perceive intellectual performance as the ability to solve problems in a structured manner, where a predefined logical solution exists. Academic instruction is thus grounded in the acquisition of analytical methods and techniques. In mathematics classrooms, deviating from explicitly detailing the calculations leading to a solution, or proposing alternative methods not covered in class, are typically considered unacceptable approaches. Students may lose points for such deviations. Responses that rely on intuition or ad hoc methods are generally evaluated as unsatisfactory.

The very components of the experimental paradigm in psychology establish the conditions for analytical reasoning to be the expected norm. Indeed, the tasks involved are artificial and typically revolve around a trap to be avoided in order to reach a rational solution. The Stroop Effect and the Müller-Lyer Illusion that we were able to address previously are basically traps, both known for inducing cognitive biases, much like calculating the probabilities of death following surgery for individuals like Mr. Roe or Mr. Smythe. Avoiding these traps involves shifting to rational thinking, while falling into them implies succumbing to patterns of thought characterized by superficiality (priming by appearances), fuzziness (non-conscious processing) and lack of rigor (a schema of knowledge influenced by subjective individual experiences). To mitigate the influence of intuition stemming from accumulated experience, experimenters focus on designing tasks that do not rely on specific prior knowledge. It is imperative to ensure that no students have an unfair advantage due to previously acquired knowledge.

However, what happens when it comes to leaving the laboratory and observing the reasoning of individuals in natural settings, particularly in work situations? In the academic context, the problems to be solved are well-mastered, well-defined problems that have undergone a uniform resolution process. A path towards the optimal solution already exists. But what about ill-defined problems that operators must solve in an uncertain environment? In such cases, does someone always have access to the "optimal solution" attainable by operators? Furthermore, what occurs when cognitive tasks are tackled by individuals with accumulated expertise? Is it conceivable to imagine intuitive thinking assisting analytical thinking, and in some cases, aided by cognitive tools? To address these questions, it is first necessary to question the assumption of the unshakable robustness of analytical thinking.

4.1. The vulnerability of analytical thinking

In everyday life, analytical thinking sometimes exhibits vulnerabilities that can result in errors. These vulnerability factors include:

– the impact of uncertainty on analytical thinking;

– the impact of short-term memory on analytical thinking;

– the effects of the individual's physiological state on their short-term memory.

4.1.1. *The impact of uncertainty on analytical thinking*

The psychologist and economist Herbert Simon (1945), Nobel laureate in economics, demonstrated that when immersed in the contingencies of reality, a decision-maker inherently possesses limited rationality. Simon thus challenged the assumption that individuals have the capacity to maximize their decision-making abilities, as posited by classical economic theory. *Decision-makers must grapple with typically ill-defined problems, where information from the environment is uncertain and incomplete.* For instance, not all available alternatives are necessarily accessible, and they often navigate dynamic environments in which data continually evolves, making definitive future projections challenging. Generally, conducting exhaustive searches for problem data, potential decision alternatives and the consequences of each alternative would require an excessively long processing time, assuming it were even feasible. Despite being equipped with highly analytical thinking capabilities, decision-makers find themselves immersed in uncertain and ambiguous environments, in which initial assumptions may prove incorrect or become outdated as the situation evolves. Moreover, when decision-makers encounter other actors involved in decision-making within their environment – such as competitors in competition – it becomes challenging to precisely ascertain the intentions and plans of these actors. Consequently, predicting the outcomes of interactions between competitors' decisions and our own decisions becomes arduous. Despite game theory's attempts to model such interactions between competing decision-makers, reality is often more complex, involving groups of individuals with diverse objectives. This complexity diminishes the efficacy of relying solely on analytical reasoning that is deemed reliable.

4.1.2. *The impact of short-term memory on analytical thinking*

Analytical thinking, relying on short-term memory, is constrained by the capacities inherent to this type of memory. Therefore, it is evident that short-term memory is limited in its ability to process information in terms of both quantity and time. If this capacity is exceeded, there is a heightened risk of information loss or distortion.

The demonstration of this limited capacity was first conducted by the psychologist George Miller (1956) in his seminal article "The magical number seven, plus or minus two: Some limits on our capacity for processing information". At the time, Miller employed the simplified model of the communication channel from Shannon's information theory to describe information processing in short-term memory. He conceptualized the stimuli perceived by an individual as inputs to a channel, with the channel's outputs corresponding to the behavioral responses elicited by these stimuli. A communication channel functioning accurately or, in other words, an effective short-term memory, would produce a response that corresponds to the presented stimuli. For instance, when presenting an image of a tree to a subject during a recognition task, we would expect the verbal response: "I see a tree". This response ultimately represents a simple linguistic recoding of a visual stimulus. Moreover, this communication channel model can also account for memorization tasks. In this scenario, the perceived information input remains stored in the channel for a certain duration before being retrieved from memory. In our example, verbal recall of the image's content occurs several hours or days after its presentation to the subject.

Miller demonstrates, based on results obtained in the laboratory, that basic tasks involving the discrimination of perceptual information and memorization are subject *to a ceiling in terms of information stored in short-term memory, with this ceiling typically around 7 +/– 2 items*. In the experiments conducted by Kaufman et al. (1949), random patterns of dots were projected onto a screen for one second. The number of points in the pattern ranged from 1 to over 200. Results indicate that subjects did not generally make recall errors on patterns containing up to five or six points. However, when presented with patterns containing more than seven points, subjects tended to have difficulty accurately identifying the number of points and relied more on approximate estimations. This limited capacity of approximately 7 units of information is also evident in word memorization mechanisms. A classic experiment in psychology, often administered to first-year students, involves the task of orally presenting a list of unrelated words, followed by recall immediately after the presentation, typically done on paper. Consistently, the average number of words recalled is around 7 plus or minus 2.

As previously discussed, short-term memory also serves as the locus of attentional resources. The prototypical model describing the functioning of attention is that of Kahneman (1973). Faced with limited attentional capacity and significant demands on attention, individuals must make choices in allocating their attentional resources among different stimuli. During tasks requiring intense concentration, the subject must allocate maximum resources to the task at hand while avoiding allocation to distractors in the surrounding environment. In situations involving multitasking, the subject must distribute attentional resources evenly. This can lead to situations in which *the operator lacks the means to deeply process a particular task due to insufficient resources*. Very superficial processing of a task indeed increases the risk of errors.

4.1.3. *The effects of the physiological state on short-term memory*

Stress and anxiety diminish the capacity to encode and retain new information in short-term memory. It is worth noting that significant fatigue in individuals can also lead to similar effects on short-term memory function.

Stress emerges due to a significant disparity between the perception of high demands arising from a task to be completed and the individual's assessment of their own capabilities to handle it (McGrath 1976; Staal 2004). This can have a major impact on the individual's attentional capacities, notably by inducing a "*tunnel effect*", characterized by a reduction in attentional focus. In this state, attention becomes restricted to primary information and tasks, while peripheral information and tasks are no longer processed. Subjectively, a task or information will be considered primary or secondary depending on its salience in the situation. If secondary elements actually had a critical role to play, the tunnel effect may lead to significant omissions. With the tunnel effect, the operator decreases the amount of information they are able to process, reducing their level of environmental exploration.

Temporal pressure is a classic stress-inducing factor. A study conducted with military decision-makers during a simulation exercise under temporal pressure demonstrates a decrease in the frequency and/or quantity of information sought by the decision-makers, as well as a decrease in accuracy in the identification of friendly or enemy submarines (Staal 2004). Noise represents another example of a stressor. It has been shown that exposure to noise can diminish the capacity to detect a signal, leading to an increase in errors. Noise amplifies the allocation of selective attention and can thus result in a tunnel effect (Staal 2004).

It is noteworthy that a stressful situation alters operators' perception of time. A study conducted with ejected fighter pilots demonstrated this phenomenon of *temporal distortion*. Twenty-eight pilots were interviewed, including questions such as whether there was a change in the apparent passage of time during ejection and, if so, what the apparent effect was. Among the sample, 75% experienced temporal distortion, while 7% were uncertain. Of those experiencing distortion, 64% reported that time seemed to slow down, while 18% felt an acceleration of time (Fair 1984; Hancock and Weaver 2005). Other findings indicate that some individuals under stress perceive events as stacking up to form a single global moment. According to Hancock and Weaver, subjective time is linked to the number of events perceived relative to real time. When many high-impact events occur in a short real-time interval, time appears to slow down – it dilates. This impression occurs when the individual's attentional resources are focused on perceiving external events. However, if the individual's attention is centered on internal concerns, they will perceive a few events occurring and thus feel that time accelerates (Hancock and Weaver 2005). The assessment of time in medical emergencies or victim care by rescuers is an important element that can disrupt operators' responsiveness to the event flow. In an emergency situation, a team may underestimate the actual elapsed time and thus overestimate their future intervention possibilities.

4.2. The power of intuitive thinking

The presence of ill-defined problems in the environment, the vulnerabilities of short-term memory, its attentional focus and the sensitivity of this memory to physiological states indicate that analytical thinking may also require support. If analytical resources can bolster intuition, there is reason to believe that intuition can compensate for the weaknesses of short-term memory and the uncertainty surrounding the decision-maker. Various findings demonstrate that it is feasible to leverage intuition to reach effective judgments and decisions.

4.2.1. *Gut feeling*

Nurses in a healthcare service have both knowledge of the health status of a patient and a relatively high level of interaction with them compared to a doctor, who primarily intervenes at key moments such as diagnosis. This position relative to the patient allows a nurse to accumulate experience in how a patient's condition evolves based on their profile, thereby developing anticipatory intuitions. *A gut feeling is the intuition that something is wrong with a patient, the feeling that their condition is deteriorating, without being able to explain the reasons for it.* This intuition can arise even when the patient's current physiological indicators are not objectively alarming. Healthcare professionals emphasize the importance of this type of intuition in their practices as an integral component of their clinical judgment and decision-making, an ability that appears to develop with experience. For instance, a nurse explains: "The longer I'm in nursing, the more my hunches are right" (Hams 2000). In the field of emergency medicine, patient assessment using intuition also plays a major role in clinical practice. An estimate suggests that intuition helps identify, in 74–87% of cases, whether the patient requires care (O'Sullivan and Schofield 2018). However, this type of intuitive judgment is often devalued pedagogically as it is considered irrational (non-analytical). Therefore, we have seen that one of the items to consider in developing clinical judgment concerns the need to find explanations to justify an emerging intuition. Intuition alone is not considered valid.

During the diagnosis of a new patient, a physician is also able to incorporate a gut feeling into their diagnosis by intuitively comparing the overall profile of this patient with profiles they typically encounter. A team of Belgian researchers collected data on consultations, carried out by general practitioners, of children with infections (Van den Bruel et al. 2014). Out of 3,890 records, 21 had been admitted to the hospital for a serious infection. At the bottom of each patient file written during the initial consultation, the physician had to justify their diagnosis by stating whether it was based on a clinical impression or a gut feeling. A clinical impression was defined as a subjective observation indicating that the illness was serious. This conclusion was based on medical history, clinical observations and a medical examination, i.e. on an analytical approach. A gut feeling was defined as an intuitive sense that something was wrong, even if the clinician was not sure of the cause. Analysis of medical records shows that the presence of a gut feeling in the physician is associated with the actual presence of a serious infection in the child, in a more significant way than the clinical impression. The analysis of the results indicates that the particular indicators associated with the emergence of a gut feeling relate to the child's general behavior (drowsiness, lack of laughter), abnormal breathing, weight loss, seizures, and relied on parental input when they indicated never having seen their child in such a state. It is noteworthy that these indicators on which the physician's intuition is built are primarily peripheral information to the key symptoms.

When considering cognitive aids, a conclusion arises: this intuitive thinking, developed on a broad and diffuse judgment regarding typical profile schemas stored in memory, may well be difficult to match with cognitive aids, designed to promote analytical decision-making. For example, Carroll (1988) studied a checklist for assessing the risk of pressure ulcers in a patient (the Norton scale). This checklist comprises five variables: the patient's physical condition, mental state, level of activity, degree of mobility and level of incontinence, with scores ranging from 1 to 4. Administering this analytical questionnaire to a group of patients, along with a questionnaire distributed to nursing staff, shows that the score on the Norton scale may sometimes indicate a low risk of pressure ulcers, while the healthcare provider intuitively judges this risk to be high, a judgment supported by years of experience.

4.2.2. *Expertise: knowledge schemas for addressing ill-defined problems*

Research in the field of human factors has long demonstrated that expertise is primarily based on intuitive, rapid and situationally adapted responses in the workplace, rather than on analytical thinking. This was evidenced by Gary Klein (1993, 2008). Contrary to intuition, Klein showed that experts continue to rely on intuitive patterns rather than analytical reasoning when dealing with new situations. According to Klein, knowledge schemas are particularly beneficial when:

– tasks to be performed are not clearly defined;

– there is a high level of uncertainty and ambiguity in the information, with some data missing;

– the situation is dynamic, with a continually evolving context;

– there is significant temporal pressure;

– there are high stakes associated with the decisions and actions to be taken;

– multiple actors are involved.

Indeed, this type of situation is challenging to process in short-term memory. However, this does not prevent expert operators from providing, in the vast majority of cases, reliable and appropriate responses to these situations, thanks to the knowledge schemas at their disposal. To describe this expert cognitive activity, Klein proposes the recognition-primed decision (RPD) model. In this model, the priming of a schema allows for the quick assimilation of a new situation to one already encountered. In cases where the operator does not directly perceive an anchoring point of a schema in the environment, they will explore the environment to search for a new cue capable of initiating a schema. Once activated, the schema may still prove to be ill-adapted to the situation. In such cases, the schema will be modified. This modification will be mentally simulated before its application, with the decision of implementation or not based on this mental test. We thus find ourselves in a cognitive process focused on prioritizing the application of a schema, whether as is or modified, rather than on analytical processing. The goal is not to inhibit a knowledge schema but to evolve it if its direct activation proves incompatible with the perceived situation. Figure 4.2 shows the application of this reasoning mode to decision-making in the paramedical field (Nibbelink and Reed 2019).

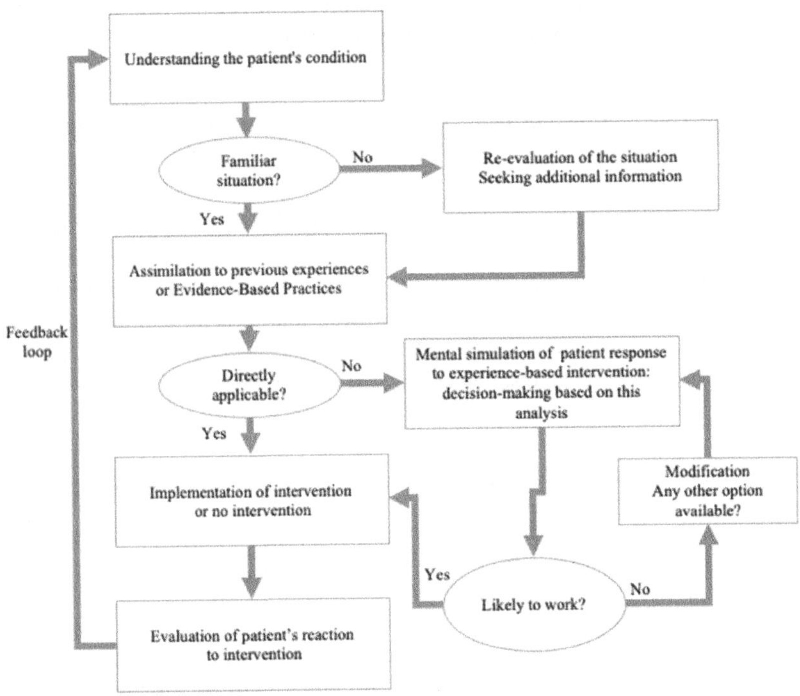

Figure 4.2. *Klein's recognition-primed decision model applied to nurses' decision-making (diagram inspired by Nibbelink and Reed (2019))*

Klein and his colleagues applied the RPD model in analyzing the cognitive activity of a team responsible for a naval anti-aircraft weapon system (Kaempf et al. 1996). This team's task is to detect flying objects, track them, identify them, discern their intentions and finally respond to them from a missile platform. The method used in the study involved conducting semi-structured interviews, guided by the critical decision method, which asks operators to recount particularly notable incidents. The interviews were recorded and coded, capturing elements related to knowledge schemas, including their goals, cues, expectations and course of action monitoring. In addition to RPD-based coding, analytical logic-based coding was performed (presence of explanations, alternative options, comparison of options for decision-making). Analysis of 14 incidents revealed that 95% of incidents were resolved based on recognition of a previous situation. Among these, 78% of decisions were based on direct priming of an end-to-end schema. Only 4% of total incidents could be classified as purely analytical logic-based.

Alongside the knowledge schemas described by Klein, there exists another typical form of intuitive schema in expertise: heuristics. Unlike the experimental approach that associates heuristics with cognitive biases, the heuristics used by experts in the world of work are instead synonymous with efficiency.

4.2.3. *Heuristics to adapt to the environment*

The work of the German psychologist Gerd Gigerenzer has rehabilitated heuristics by highlighting their highly adaptive nature. Gigerenzer defines a *heuristic* as "a strategy that ignores part of the information, with the goal of making decisions more quickly, frugally, and/or accurately than more complex methods" (Gigerenzer and Gaissmaier 2011). This definition implies that heuristics can sometimes outperform analytical reasoning.

An anecdote mentioned by Gigerenzer's team (Hafenbrädl et al. 2016) concerns the management of a financial portfolio. In 1990, Harry Markowitz received the Nobel Prize in Economics for his theoretical work on the optimal allocation of assets, particularly regarding the choice between saving for retirement or immediately investing in the stock market. Markowitz had demonstrated that there was an optimal portfolio that maximized returns for retirement funds. However, for his own retirement, Markowitz did not use his optimization model. Instead he relied on a simple heuristic, which involved evenly distributing money across a certain number of investment funds (the 1/N rule, with N being the number of funds). Studies have shown that this heuristic is frequently used in the population. Finance researchers criticized this behavior as simplistic. However, a subsequent rigorous study compared the results of 12 asset allocation optimization strategies in seven situations. The results showed that despite the high level of sophistication of some of these strategies in terms of probability calculation, none of the 12 strategies yielded results as good as those obtained with the 1/N heuristic (DeMiguel et al. 2009).

Heuristics circumvent the manipulation of complex domain laws, principles and computational rules. Moreover, they help to constrain the combinatorial explosion induced by analyzing a situation comprising multiple variables that interact with each other. Here are some examples:

– *The recognition heuristic*: when faced with a choice between two interpretations of the same situation, this heuristic involves selecting the alternative that is most familiar. Johnson and Raab (2003) demonstrated that experienced handball players can effectively rely on the first alternative that comes to mind when deciding which technical move to execute during a match (a strategy called "take the first").

– *The one-clever-cue heuristic*: it involves considering only one specific item of information to base a decision on. For instance, when baseball players chase after the ball, research has demonstrated that they adjust their speed based on a single cue: maintaining a constant angle between their viewpoint and the ball.

– *The trade-off heuristic*: this strategy involves facing the uncertainty of potential effects from multiple alternatives by opting for a compromise to avoid the negative consequences associated with a radical choice for a single alternative (e.g. the 1/N distribution choice).

– *The fast and frugal tree*: this heuristic involves dealing with a high number of cues by prioritizing the exploration of key cues in a specific order. At each cue (or question about that cue), a binary decision of "yes/no" is made to proceed further along the tree or stop at a final conclusion (Martignon et al. 2008; Jenny et al. 2013; Hafenbrädl et al. 2016). The utility of fast and frugal trees in the healthcare field and their integration with cognitive aids has been demonstrated by Green and Mehr (1997) and Gigerenzer and Kurzenhäuzer (2005). When a patient arrives at the emergency room with chest pain, the decision is either to send the patient directly to a coronary care unit or to keep them under observation. Researchers studied this decision-making process under two conditions: free decision-making by the physician (condition A) and decision-making with a cognitive aid presenting potential clinical scenarios and probabilities of occurrence (condition B). The study protocol followed an ABAB design, alternating between the two conditions over time with the same physicians. The results indicate that under condition A, where the decision is based solely on the physician's judgment, admission to the emergency unit includes 90% false positives – patients who did not have serious risks but were still sent to the emergency care unit. With the table presenting probabilities, this false positive rate drops to approximately 60%, demonstrating the value of this (analytical) cognitive aid for better adjustment to the actual severity of encountered situations. However, it is also observed that in subsequent conditions, with or without aid, the percentage of false positives remains approximately 60%, even when physicians no longer have the cognitive aid with them. According to the authors, it is not conceivable that physicians have retained all the data listed in the document; what they retained is the fundamental structure governing the presented data; somewhat akin to the formal grammar learned by participants in Reber's implicit learning experiment. Mentally, they constructed from this document a representation resembling a fast and frugal tree.

This hypothesis led the authors to devise such a decision tree, which accounts for a hierarchical classification of cases. With the following three criteria prioritized among them: a change in the patient's ECG, dominant chest pain and other associated factors related to history. The results demonstrate that this decision tree is more sensitive than a logistic regression-type statistical model. Patients who are genuinely in critical condition are directed to the emergency room. The decision tree is also more specific, meaning it generates fewer false positives than the statistical model or the intuition of the physician, despite being much simpler and based on less data than the statistical model. According to Gigerenzer, this superiority of the fast and frugal tree over a mathematical model lies in the fact that it directly reflects the very structure of the information from the environment. In this context, he refers to ecological rationality adjusted to the constraints present in the environment, whereas the statistical model is a post hoc construction based on the extraction of collected data.

According to Gigerenzer, heuristics face unjustified criticism that leads to undervaluing their adaptive qualities. These criticisms include:

– the notion that they produce less satisfactory results compared to sophisticated analytical strategies. In reality, optimization based on analytical grounds is often impossible or very challenging due to uncontrollable variability in many situations;

– the belief that our psyche relies on heuristics due to our limited cognitive capacities. Gigerenzer argues that it is the probabilistic nature of the environment, coupled with our cognitive limitations, that prompts the development of heuristics;

– the misconception that heuristics are only used for routine, low-stakes decisions. However, heuristics are observed even in critical decisions, such as those made by emergency physicians during diagnosis;

– the assumption that heuristics are characteristic of individuals with lower intellectual capacities. Research on the relationship between intellectual abilities and heuristic usage shows no significant correlation between the prevalence of heuristics and IQ;

– the idea that individuals with more information and sophisticated cognitive processes make better decisions. Gigerenzer demonstrates that decisions made in uncertain environments can sometimes be beneficial precisely because they ignore certain information that may ultimately disrupt reasoning;

– the belief that heuristics cannot be evaluated. Gigerenzer illustrates that it is possible to computer model heuristics and demonstrate their effectiveness.

Knowledge schemas and heuristics serve the purpose of making decisions based on stable patterns extracted from the environment – pieces of information that remain constant despite the apparent variability of situations. This expert knowledge helps to alleviate the internal burden of processing new information in short-term memory. Heuristics also provide a means to navigate challenging working conditions. An anesthesiologist recounted that when working night shifts and experiencing significant fatigue, he intentionally relied on simple yet reliable heuristics rather than engaging in complex reasoning sensitive to the effects of fatigue.

4.2.4. *Chunks to surpass the capacity of short-term memory*

While Miller (1958) wrote a seminal article delineating the confines of short-term memory, the concluding segment of this very article also served as an opportunity to demonstrate the potential for surpassing these boundaries. While short-term storage capacity hovers around seven units for information lacking interrelations, this capacity substantially increases when individuals discern connections that enable the consolidation of information units. These consolidated units, termed "chunks", once mentally formulated by the individual, facilitate the retrieval from memory not of approximately seven basic items (words, numbers), but rather of groupings, each comprising up to seven items. Consequently, the cumulative volume of stored information can become considerable. *To form a chunk, it is "enough" to identify a relationship that amalgamates several ostensibly independent items into a single cohesive unit of information.* Once amalgamated, these items can be encoded in long-term memory and retrieved via their shared address. Such relationships may vary in nature, provided they enable the consolidation and retrieval of information (phonetic proximity, lexical congruence, logical sequence, etc.). For instance, communication protocol acronyms rely on lexical chunks. Schemas within long-term memory serve as a particularly potent framework for the formation of chunks.

The ability to develop chunks based on expertise was demonstrated by Gobet (1998) in an experimental task but within a domain characterized by genuine expertise, namely, the game of chess. Players with varying levels of expertise were tasked with memorizing the arrangement of pieces on chessboards. Some boards displayed pieces arranged in typical configurations reflective of ongoing games, while others presented random arrangements. The findings indicate that while recall performance remains relatively stable for random layouts across participants, irrespective of their chess proficiency, this performance steadily improves with players' expertise levels for realistic configurations. As players become more proficient, they leverage their expertise to cultivate chunks, thereby enhancing the retrieval of information from memory.

Knowledge schemas not only guide the memorization of information but also its recognition. In a task involving the identification of information within a medical image, we enlisted 25 participants (five neurosurgeons, 10 medical interns, 10 medical imaging engineers) to examine the contents of brain images from a patient with a brain lesion (Morineau et al. 2013). The 82 pieces of information provided to participants were previously categorized by an expert based on their level of abstraction, ranging from concrete details like cortical surface (gyri) to highly abstract information such as the perception of lesion extraction strategy within the image. Abstract information inherently encompassed a significant amount of basic information (chunks). Participants could classify their identification as direct, indirect (requiring analytical effort) or absent. Results indicate the particularly pronounced impact of expertise level, especially in perceiving units of information containing a wealth of elementary data. For instance, the information "tumor extraction strategy" is perceived within the image by all neurosurgeons, with 40% perceiving it directly and 60% indirectly. In contrast, no intern or imaging engineer perceives it directly. 40% of interns and 20% of imaging engineers report perceiving it indirectly in the image.

These findings demonstrate that experts, when confronted with challenges in real-world environments, exhibit capabilities such as intuition, activation of relevant schemas and making judgments and decisions based on heuristics and chunks. Given the advantages of intuitive thinking, could it not be considered a resource that could be harnessed through cognitive aids?

4.3. Slowness and risks in accessing intuitive resources unaided

Finding implicit knowledge schemas independently, without external assistance, is indeed feasible, but it involves a lengthy and risky process. This process corresponds to the mechanism of skill acquisition by transforming declarative knowledge, processed in short-term memory, into procedural knowledge processed in long-term memory (Anderson 1992). It is widely accepted in ergonomics that acquiring expertise requires at least 10 years of practice in a specific field. Acquiring a particular procedural schema (approximately 100 hours of practice on average) involves a learning process that is not only protracted but also error-prone, as error is an inherent component of learning. Learning occurs through trial and error and, in this regard, risk management policies aimed at systematically eliminating errors diminish the possibility of organizational learning.

To elucidate the roles of the "time" and "risk-taking" factors associated with learning, we can turn to the research conducted by Bokhari et al. (2011) regarding the learning curve in the adoption of the da Vinci Surgical System in the United States. Using a retrospective database comprising 50 surgeries, the authors tracked the evolution of interaction time between the surgeon and the instrument during surgical procedures. Their findings delineate three distinct phases of development. The initial phase, spanning from the first robot-assisted surgery to the 15th, demonstrates a gradual reduction in the time required by the surgeon to perform operations, indicating the surgeon's progress in the mastery of the robot. Phase 2, spanning the 15th to the 25th surgery, exhibits a stabilization of surgical duration, signifying proficiency in robot operation. Phases 1 and 2 typically depict a standard learning curve. However, the authors also identify an unforeseen third phase, spanning the 25th to the 50th surgery. In this final phase they note, counterintuitively, a decline in performance manifested by a continuous increase in surgery duration.

To comprehend this regression, we must take into account the factor of "risk-taking" in surgery. Initially, the surgeries performed with the robot were for simple procedures, aiming to mitigate errors with critical implications for the patient. It was only after mastering the robot (phase 2) that it was used in more complex procedures (phase 3). Consequently, surgery duration increased again due to the inherent complexity of the operative procedures made feasible by the now-mastered robot.

Measuring learning goes beyond mere quantification. The transition from a declarative mode of knowledge to a procedural one represents a qualitative shift in information processing. Surgeons encounter a novel perceptual setup, wherein they must substitute tactile and kinesthetic cues, typically relied upon during tissue manipulation, with visual indicators. Additionally, they must mentally visualize the position of robotic instruments without direct scene visualization. When dealing with human subjects, learning thus necessitates both time and the management of associated risks inherent in skill assimilation. Given the arduous journey towards mastering knowledge schemas, could we not seek support in cognitive aids to facilitate swift access to intuition, patterns, heuristics and chunks?

4.4. Access to intuition thanks to cognitive aids

While cognitive aids that facilitate analytical thinking primarily serve to elucidate knowledge, those oriented towards intuitive thinking must logically, on the contrary, provide schemas containing implicit knowledge.

This implicit knowledge enables the provision of rapid responses that require minimal mental resources. Figure 4.3 shows a collection of tools capable of transforming information from a mere list into resources that facilitate intuition, rather than analytical resources as previously discussed. While not exhaustive, the following instruments, which convey knowledge schemas, can be mentioned.

– *Mnemonic devices*: these are methods of condensing information in a meaningful manner to facilitate memorization, or, in other words, a way of forming information chunks. Acronyms provide easily memorable addresses. For instance, the ABCDE (Airway, Breathing, Circulation, Disability, Exposure) emergency medical protocol offers guidance on evaluating essential patient functions in critical situations (respiratory tract, oxygenation, circulatory system, nervous system, hemorrhage or trauma). It is important to distinguish the acronym of a communication procedure or protocol from its content, which pertains to an analytical structuring of knowledge.

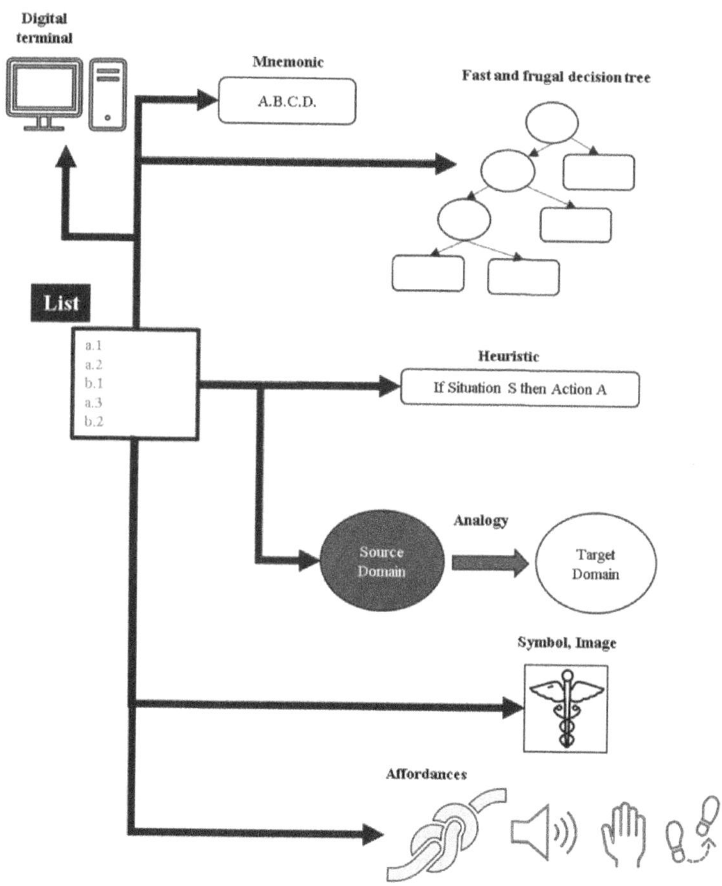

Figure 4.3. *Cognitive gateways facilitating intuitive thinking from a list of items*

– *Fast and frugal trees and other forms of heuristics*: fast and frugal trees make it possible to avoid explanation of all variables in decision-making, as discussed previously. An example of a fast and frugal tree designed as a disseminable and shareable cognitive aid is the "START" procedure in the field of damage control, used during the triage of casualties in hazardous situations such as disasters, attacks or war zones, where time constraints are severe, medical resources are limited and numerous victims are present. In this decision tree, the initial criterion is to assess if the victim can walk unaided; if not, their breathing is observed. If breathing is compromised, their radial pulse is checked. If the pulse is weak, the person's responsiveness to a simple request is evaluated (Luan et al. 2011). Heuristics are simpler decision-making formulas than decision trees, constructed on the basis of conditions that prompt a decision (the "if… then…" rule). They encapsulate the essential and sufficient cues for triggering an adaptive response.

– *Analogy*: analogies implicitly facilitate the understanding of a "target" domain that is still unfamiliar, drawing from a "source" domain that is already known. It involves leveraging an existing mental representation to swiftly and easily develop another. For instance, likening the structure of an atom with its electrons to planets revolving around the Sun serves to elucidate the concept. Merely suggesting that the atom's structure "resembles" that of the solar system conveys implicit inferences such as the spherical nature of objects and rotation around a larger central entity. The power of analogy lies in its ability to provide a cohesive set of conclusions about the state of a target domain that has not yet been mastered by the listener. The concept of the Vortex (Chrimes 2016) to describe patient oxygenation progression is rooted in the principle of analogy (source domain: the vortex; target domain: oxygenation).

– *Symbols and images*: the symbolism of colors, icons, images and animations enables concrete representation of information within context. These signifiers diminish the need for extensive textual explanation. Such formats for presenting information bridge abstract thinking with tangible properties (affordances) that, through their appearance, can readily guide the operator's actions.

– *Affordances*: while originally belonging to the natural environment, humans have engineered artificial environments that introduce new affordances. Rasmussen (1986) and Norman (1988) were among the first to recognize the potential of affordance in ergonomics. Designers who successfully create affordant objects enable ergonomic solutions, as the objects' usability is inherently facilitated by the immediate perception of their properties. The embodiment of information in a physical medium facilitates the construction of affordances. The practice of tying a knot in a handkerchief serves as a prototypical cognitive aid, offering an affordance designed to assist in information retrieval. In Central America, the Incas developed a system for recording knowledge, not through writing, but via systems of cords known as "quipus". In work settings, affordances can engage operators' various sensory channels: visible object properties, alarms, tactile and haptic feedback from objects, as well as spatial zones defining the workspace, which provide perceptible affordances during movement.

Fuchs et al. (2021) proposed designing an emergency cart highly guided by affordances (shapes, colors) to enhance the differentiation between various syringes and drug categories. The proposed cart is structured to mitigate the disorder sometimes observed in medical carts and prevent overstocking. Disorder and overstocking contribute to informational noise. Figure 4.4 shows a segment of this pediatric emergency cart, focusing on the arrangement of laryngoscopes.

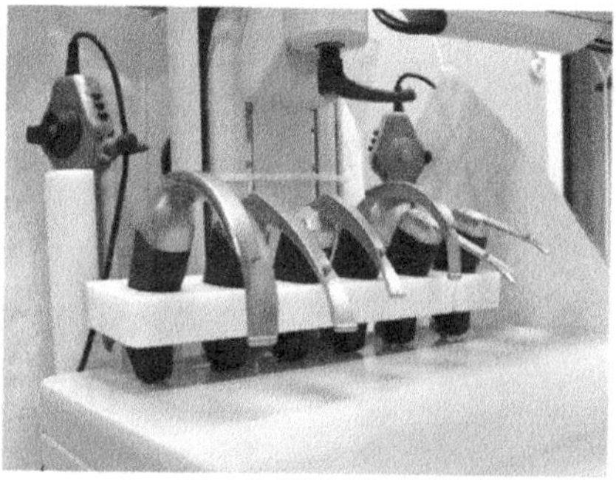

Figure 4.4. *Facilitating affordances for identifying laryngoscopes (direct perception–action, directly visible blade sizes) on a prototype medical cart (source: free reproduction from Fuchs et al. (2021)). For a color version of this figure, see www.iste.co.uk/morineau/cognitive.zip*

Indeed, this arrangement, which may seem inconspicuous at first glance, embodies two particularly helpful properties: 1) the instruments are both directly perceivable and graspable (not concealed in a drawer); 2) the instruments are organized to facilitate the selection of a blade size, an important consideration based on the physical characteristics of the child.

– *Digital terminals*: a calculator, a phone application or a computer containing decision support software are examples of digital terminals that support a function that would otherwise have required a long period of learning to achieve the same level of performance. However, for a digital terminal to truly facilitate intuitive thinking, it must be ergonomic. In this regard, the "software" part will be designed by exploiting other possible formats to facilitate the implicit, such as analogy (the virtual desktop of a computer is now inspired by the real desktop), symbols and images (icons, graphical representation of stored data), or even affordances (direct manipulation of virtual objects through a touchscreen, or even immersion in a virtual world).

Digital terminals also provide access to affordances that would otherwise be inaccessible. Medical imaging systems and miniaturized cameras used to guide surgical procedures enable physicians to access affordances hidden within the human body. With these technologies, organs inside the body become directly perceptible, which represents a significant advancement for diagnosis and medical procedures. The videolaryngoscope is an example of a device that makes the perception of the trachea more accessible during intubation. The challenge of the procedure is to avoid the adjacent natural passage, the esophagus, which leads to the stomach. The laryngoscope helps facilitate the exposure of the trachea during the insertion of the tube. Compared to a traditional laryngoscope, a videolaryngoscope additionally features a miniature camera located on the blade tip and a small screen (Figure 4.5).

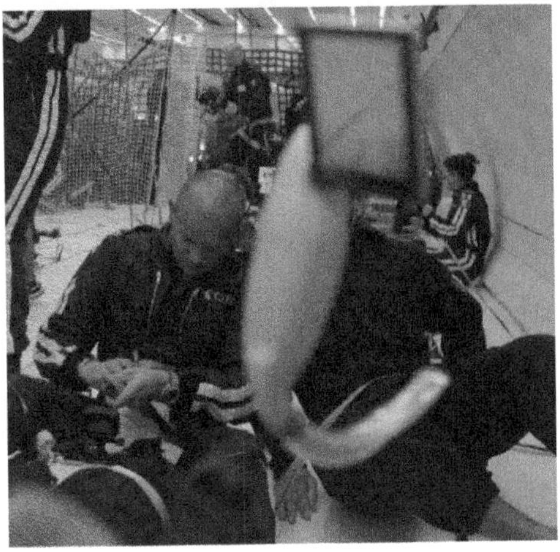

Figure 4.5. *Simulated intubation on a mannequin during parabolic flight (microgravity), with a videolaryngoscope in the foreground. Photo credits: Novespace/AirZeroG. For a color version of this figure, see www.iste.co.uk/morineau/cognitive.zip*

The contribution of the videolaryngoscope as a tool in medical procedures has been demonstrated in a study comparing both experts and novices under normal and extreme intubation conditions (Stark et al. 2020). Three experienced physicians (with over 1,000 intubations) and three novices (with fewer than 10 intubations) participated in an experiment involving intubating a mannequin using either a traditional laryngoscope or a videolaryngoscope, both on Earth and aboard an aircraft performing parabolic flights to simulate weightlessness in space for 20 seconds, an extreme condition akin to patient care aboard a space station. The results indicate that experts outperform novices regardless of the intubation conditions; however, in weightlessness, novices improve their performance when using the videolaryngoscope compared to the traditional laryngoscope. Under these weightless conditions, their performance does not significantly differ from that of experts in the same conditions. Therefore, the videolaryngoscope facilitates a performance level close to that of experts and makes it possible to cope with extreme working conditions. This device serves as support for both factors involved in a cognitive system: the individual with their own expertise and the environment, which constrains activity.

Note that digital terminals can serve as supports for both analytical and intuitive thinking, similar to basic supports like paper sheets. Both analytical tables and symbolic images can be displayed on a digital screen.

4.5. Conclusion

In academic circles, intellectual performance is typically viewed as following the path laid out by logical-mathematical norms to enable effective problem-solving. When intuitive thinking predominates, it consequently implies irrational reasoning, susceptible to appearances and subject to cognitive biases. Intuition must then be replaced by analytical thinking. While this approach may hold validity in a classroom setting, it becomes less evident when considering cognition in natural environments in which constraints that have not been artificially constructed constitute the data of the problems to be solved. In daily life, problems are mostly ill-defined, often dynamic, with sometimes no clear-cut answers held by anyone, or even potentially accessible.

In such contexts, the reference point ceases to be an ideal standard. Instead, knowledge and skills developed through acquired experience serve as the reference. However, as observed, expertise primarily resides within the intuitive system. It relies on a gradual process of extracting regularities from the environment. In the words of Gigerenzer, this is termed ecological rationality, which is grounded in cognitive schemas, heuristics and affordances. This expertise enables individuals to address the constraints of a situation without delving into analytical reasoning, which could be time-consuming, mentally taxing, sensitive to stress and fatigue, and hence prone to errors due to haste or breakdowns in the lengthy chain of inferences required.

When expertise cannot be directly implemented due to resource constraints (such as time for learning), cognitive aids aimed at facilitating responses to a situation can be considered. This will be the role of assistive devices providing access to cognitive schemas, including easily retrievable acronyms, frugal trees, shared heuristics within a team, analogical connections between well-mastered and new domains, guiding action through symbols and easily understandable images, affordances embedded in manipulable objects or the use of technology enabling direct access to otherwise concealed affordances. Through these tools, the novice's performance can approach that of an expert. However, it is important to note that replacing the lengthy process of acquiring expertise with cognitive aids may not always be feasible or desirable. The aim is to support access to expertise rather than replace it entirely. Otherwise, there is a risk of reverting to a static perspective, wherein knowledge storage is divided between external and internal cognitions. A cognitive system is a dynamic interaction fundamentally involving, at a minimum, an individual and an environment.

Therefore, the concept of a cognitive gateway allows for a deeper understanding of cognitive aids by prompting consideration of the types of knowledge to be supplemented to operators, reinforcing their response to the demands of a task or a degraded work context. Being able to envision a device that facilitates access either to intuitive or analytical thinking enables exploration of the full spectrum of human cognition resources to find assistance solutions. As psychologist Maurice Reuchlin argued, each individual's reasoning in a given situation is not uniform but *vicarious* (Reuchlin 1978). Faced with the expected vulnerabilities of system 1 (intuitive), we look for aids providing analytical thinking. Conversely, when faced with the anticipated vulnerabilities of system 2 (analytical), we design aids that foster intuitive thinking. Cognitive aid acts as a two-way gateway.

On the contrary, this gateway can be established between resources internal to the same individual (such as notes taken on a sheet of paper in the healthcare provider's gown, enabling them to articulate observations through writing) or between resources distributed among several individuals (such as a patient management algorithm displayed in a department). This latter scenario is easily conceivable because a cognitive aid is a shareable tool within a community. Within a team, cognitive aids can be exchanged, much like sharing best practices. Furthermore, in this context of sharing, other actors besides the healthcare providers themselves will find opportunities to intervene, viewing support for assistance as a means to contribute to activity (such as adding managerial instructions to the displayed medical algorithm). This is what we will explore next.

5

Routing Prescribed Tasks to Support the Actual Activity

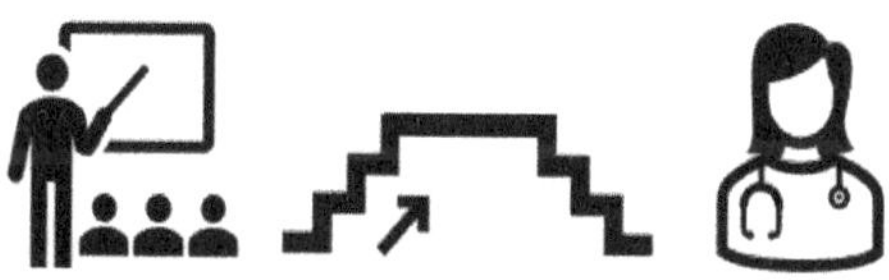

Figure 5.1. *Prescribers (hospital executives, domain experts) can transmit task descriptions to healthcare providers via cognitive aids*

In a hospital in Brazil, the conflict between management and hospital service agents responsible for bio-cleaning cannot be resolved (Idal Sznelwar et al. 2003). Some of these agents suffer from poisoning and take sick leave. Faced with these cases of poisoning, management emphasizes the importance of adhering to cleaning instructions and using the provided products. However, it is observed that some staff members do not comply with these instructions. They believe that the provided products are not effective enough and thus take it upon themselves to create their own disinfectants, often using personal recipes involving hot water and various mixtures, which can emit toxic fumes. In summary, there is a disparity between the prescribed task, which involves following cleaning instructions provided by management, and the actual activity, which diverges significantly and dangerously from these prescribed tasks.

Francophone ergonomics and work psychology have long demonstrated the almost systematic nature of observable discrepancies between instructions and actual activity. Notably, not all observed deviations in the field lead to adverse events. However, the recurring presence of deviations indicates that contextual constraints compel behaviors to move away from the instructions formalized in documents. Researcher Erik Hollnagel (2018) recently revitalized these concepts in anglophone literature, referring to "work as imagined" (prescribed task) and "work as done" (actual activity). While some deviations may constitute positive adaptations to real-world constraints, others may introduce error sources. René Amalberti (2013), a specialist in human factors in health and former advisor to the French National Authority for Health, identifies various strategies in hospital care activities, characterized by their degree of non-compliance with prescribed tasks.

– Type A strategies: all tasks are executed in accordance with recommended protocols, yielding expected outcomes. In the French hospital sector, this type of strategy represents only 40% of interventions.

– Type B strategies: these involve adaptations of protocols potentially leading to minor adverse events. According to the author, this accounts for 50% of medical interventions.

– Type C strategies: this involves a cautious approach where ideal conditions for task execution are awaited before commencement. For instance, postponing surgery. However, the risk lies in the potential negative consequences of activity postponement. This strategy is estimated to apply to 10% of interventions.

– Type D strategies: the violation of protocols is significant enough to trigger critical events, with severe repercussions for patients, occurring in 0.1–0.5% of interventions.

To prevent these hazardous deviations, it is possible to implement countermeasures (Reason 2000). These measures can be constructive, such as prevention campaigns and staff retraining periods. Alternatively, countermeasures can also be punitive, involving disciplinary or legal actions identification of involved parties and assigning blame. Another approach to countermeasures is the development of new procedures or the revision of existing ones to refine instructions provided to staff, making them more easily applicable in real-world situations and thereby avoiding risky deviations. In the healthcare domain, it is important to note that knowledge evolves, and the inadequacy of activities may stem from care guidelines that are outdated and suboptimal in content.

Ideally, the prescribed task should function as a psychological instrument, capable of being internalized by staff and, in certain contexts, providing genuine assistance in their work. A particular challenge in the hospital setting lies in formulating prescribed tasks due to the existence of two types of prescribers for healthcare providers: domain experts who establish clinical guidelines and institutional managers who formalize work instructions. With two sets of prescribed tasks in play, there is theoretically twice the risk of observing discrepancies between the task and actual activity.

Considering task requirements within the framework of cognitive aids involves questioning how to construct and route these prescriptions in a manner that prevents critical deviations during implementation in context. *In other words, cognitive gateways can also serve as intermediaries between expected tasks and observable practices in the field.*

5.1. Guidelines from domain experts

In response to the variability of practices, health guidelines aim to assist clinicians by providing a healthcare approach that is both uniform and effective. These guidelines endeavor to be based on the gold standard of practices, which are validated by the most recent empirical evidence. To achieve this objective, it is necessary to standardize healthcare practices according to those recognized as the best by the community, while also transitioning from the concept of guidelines to that of cognitive aids.

5.1.1. *Standardizing healthcare practices*

Guidelines are constructed based on empirical findings, fostering consensus within expert committees. They also serve to raise awareness of practices with questionable outcomes and potential contraindications (Zuiderent-Jerak et al. 2011; Wieringa et al. 2018). While guideline recommendations primarily stem from results obtained in experimental settings and meta-analyses of research studies, they draw upon various sources. In instances where scientific evidence is lacking or conflicting, insights and experiences from healthcare providers and recipients contribute to knowledge (Wieringa et al. 2018). However, developing best practices requires a rigorous methodology. Internationally, the Institute of Medicine in the United States (noted for its report on medical errors) pioneered the establishment of a framework for defining clinical indications. This effort led to the formation of an international working group on clinical guidelines known as the "Guidelines International Network" (GIN). The GIN group conducts international monitoring of the benefits and challenges associated with guideline implementation (Perkins et al. 2021). Table 5.1 outlines the conditions necessary for an expert group to develop guidelines (Quaseem et al. 2012).

Once the guidelines have been developed by the expert committee, the next step is to ensure their implementation in practice, rather than allowing them to remain merely as textual descriptions of best practices. This transition from prescribed task to actual activity is where deviations may arise. However, it is evident that numerous contextual factors can hinder the application of recommendations. Many studies on guideline implementation in healthcare services demonstrate various barriers that limit their actual impact on improving the quality of healthcare. In a literature review on this subject, Correa et al. (2020) provide a synthesis of both barriers and facilitators identified in healthcare settings regarding best practices. We propose to categorize these positive and negative factors based on whether they relate to individual healthcare professionals, the broader healthcare team or the content of the guidelines themselves.

Components	Description
Composition of the guideline development group	Establish a group comprising diverse and relevant stakeholders, including healthcare professionals, methodologists, subject matter experts and patients
Decision-making processes	Detail the process used to reach consensus among panel members and, if required, secure approval from supporting organizations
Conflicts of interest	Identify potential financial and non-financial conflicts of interest. This document should also outline how conflicts were identified, recorded and resolved
Topics of the guidelines	Specify the objectives and topics addressed
Methods	Clearly and comprehensively describe the methods used for guideline development
Review of evidence	Use systematic review methods of evidence and rely on scientific evidence concerning benefits, risks and, if possible, costs
Evaluation of evidence and recommendations	Use an evaluation system to communicate the quality and reliability of evidence and the value of recommendations
Peer consultation	Have recommendations reviewed by an external agency before publication
Expiration of guidelines	Provide an expiration date to ensure guideline updates
Financial support and sponsorship	Disclose financial support for both the evidence review and recommendations

Table 5.1. *Essential components for refining guidelines, according to the Guidelines International Network (adapted from Quaseem et al. (2012))*

– At the individual level: professionals often encounter challenges in accessing the necessary conditions to assimilate existing guidelines in their field. Healthcare providers may lack awareness of the existence of guidelines and the procedures for locating them. Even when guidelines are known, healthcare providers often lack the time to study and implement them. Similarly, patients face difficulties in accessing recommendations, and if they are aware of them but lack a thorough understanding, they may disrupt their relationship with the physician.

– At the team level: the absence of a leader capable of establishing priorities and managing the implementation of directives within the team is a significant barrier.

Similarly, challenges in teamwork, lack of coordination, recurrent disagreements among colleagues and unclear delineation of responsibilities do not foster the sharing of the latest recommendations. For guidelines to become a genuine external resource available to a team to enhance their work, clear leadership is necessary to set objectives and cultivate enthusiasm within the group. It is worth noting that multidisciplinary teams facilitate this dynamic, along with unwavering support from hospital administration.

– At the content level of the guidelines: guidelines themselves can contain barriers to their implementation. These barriers can be classified based on the criteria of accessibility, trust and reliability that we have used for cognitive aids. Accessibility can be challenging. Healthcare providers sometimes complain about the lack of clarity in the instructions. They may appear too rigid and conflict with usual practices within the team. They do not align with everyday tasks. To reduce these obstacles, healthcare providers expect documents to be in a concise and simple format, with brochures for patients if necessary. Guidelines should require the least possible additional resources for implementation. Lack of trust and doubts about the reliability of guidelines are sometimes observed in services. Some professionals believe that the guidelines are incorrect or insufficiently justified. Professionals would like end-users to be more involved in their development, implementation and field testing. By not meeting the criteria of accessibility, trust and reliability, guidelines are not well-positioned to integrate directly into the cognitive system of a healthcare team and its work environment. If the document manages to reach the service, it risks ending up in a drawer.

For such a document to be truly effective, it must not only be read and shared but also adapted onto various platforms to ensure it is ergonomic in diverse clinical settings. It must be acknowledged that guidelines are not directly applicable; they require a prior "translation", a reformulation through documents where information is filtered, recoded and reformatted to accommodate the information processing constraints across different contexts. The aim is to align the guidelines with real-world clinical activity, effectively transforming them into practical work aids.

5.1.2. *Transitioning from guidelines to cognitive aids*

Figure 5.2 provides an overview of the various generic phases within the clinical activity of a healthcare team. At the core of the figure lies patient management, which is central to clinical activity. This phase involves interventions with the patient, collaboration among healthcare providers, resolution of basic or complex issues, and monitoring of progress in patient care. Translated guidelines aimed at facilitating intervention and collaboration during patient care may include structured requests, verbalizations synchronized with actions, a whiteboard or a digital screen.

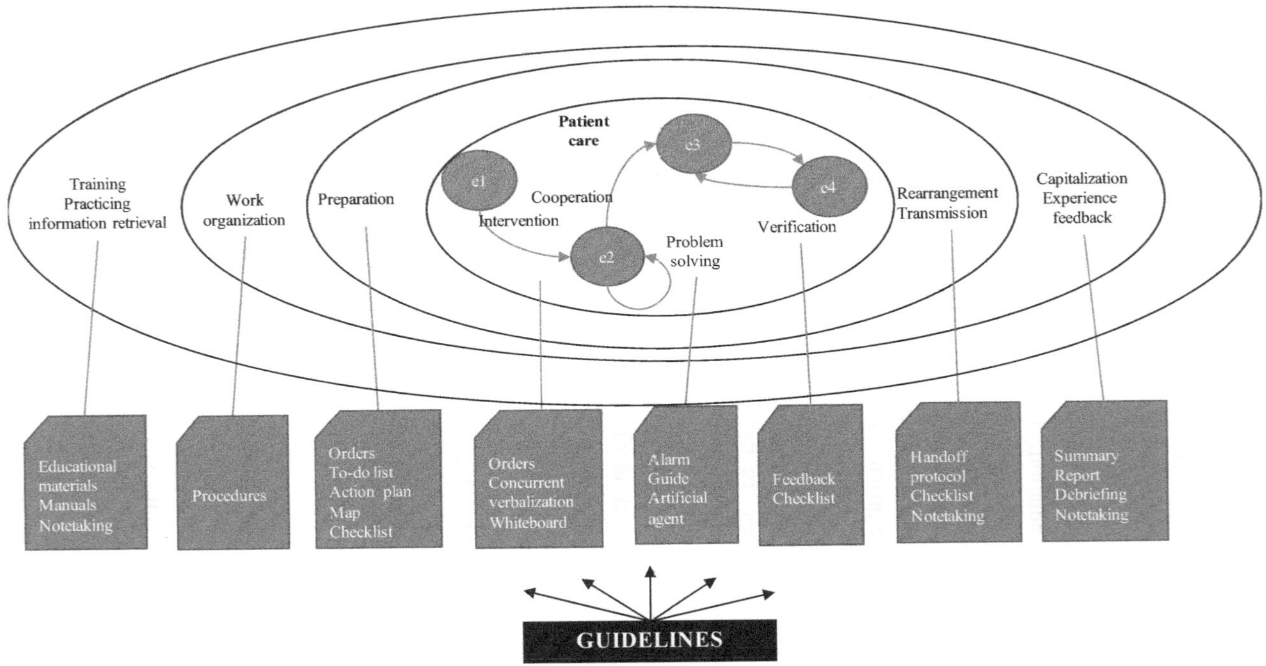

Figure 5.2. *Guidelines integrated into dedicated cognitive aids for various stages of clinical activity in a care team*

Problem solving can be facilitated by alarms, guides, an artificial agent performing calculations or information searches in a database. Progress verification will involve team exchanges and the use of a checklist. To address the common temporal pressure within healthcare, these cognitive aids will selectively present directive content, prioritize oral communication and rely on automated systems for reliable and swift *information processing*.

Around patient management, we find upstream the *phase of training and practicing* for the teams. Educational materials and manuals will present the guidelines of the domain in detail. An application software such as "DansMaBlouse", seen previously, will enable the compilation of documents including note-taking. Having access to this data on a smartphone allows for continuous use throughout the different stages of care. The *phase of organizing work* allows teams to anticipate everyone's roles and necessary equipment, with documents outlining the protocol's main points, such as a flowchart. The *preparation phase* will be based on instructions given to team members, such as remembering to communicate clearly or signaling when everyone is ready to receive instructions (Perkins et al. 2021). To-do lists, action plans, a plan showing the positions each person should have around the patient and a checklist for verifying available equipment will provide support for activity during the preparation phase.

Following patient care, the *rearrangement* of the room to prepare it for a new patient or the *protocol* phase if teams are alternating can be facilitated using a checklist and an oral protocol. The final phase involves *capitalizing* on past events to enhance future care through feedback on experience. Paper documents and debriefings with team members will serve as the means for this.

Clearly, this diagram is not exhaustive in terms of the cognitive aids that may be involved. Instead, it aims to illustrate that guidelines must adapt to various usage contexts. By analyzing the constraints and information needs of these contexts, we can determine the content to display and specify how to communicate it. Simply placing the guideline manual on a shelf in the department and leaving it there is not sufficient. For instance, the 2021 Neonatal Resuscitation Guidelines constitute Chapter 8 of the European Resuscitation Council Resuscitation Guidelines (Perkins et al. 2021). This chapter, structured into 25 pages and 17 sections of text, requires careful reading in a calm environment, such as an office, or before preparing a training session. However, it is worth noting that the editors have endeavored to ease knowledge assimilation by introducing psychological aids, such as a list of key information for resuscitation (top message) and an algorithm summarizing the care process. These presentations aim to bridge the gap between the lengthy original text and the constraints of real-world use.

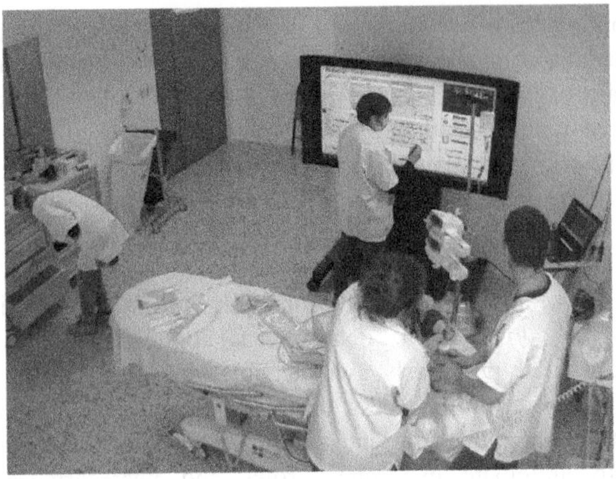

Figure 5.3. *Use of a large touchscreen displaying instructions during a training session for newborn resuscitation on a simulator (source: University of Southern Brittany, LP3C Laboratory, reproduction authorized by Excense and IFPS Vannes). For a color version of this figure, see www.iste.co.uk/morineau/cognitive.zip*

The ideal approach is to *completely rethink guidelines based on the context and the type of assistance possible*. Figure 5.3 shows the use of a cognitive aid prototype in a simulation room designed to convey guidelines during newborn resuscitation (Boulanger et al. 2021). These instructions are displayed on a large touchscreen positioned in the delivery room. A healthcare provider, with the status of supervisor, interacts with the information system, guiding caregivers through checklist items during each phase of care, prompting them to verbalize their actions aloud. This device serves not only as a visual memory aid but also initiates real-time verbalizations concurrent with actions, fostering enhanced situational awareness sharing within the team.

In addition to guidelines from experts, task requirements are the managers' responsibility in a medical or healthcare institution.

5.2. Instructions from hospital managers

As highlighted in the introduction to this chapter, the hospital domain exhibits the unique characteristic of a bipartite authority structure (or even a tripartite structure if we distinguish between the medical and paramedical bodies). This includes the authority of caregivers, expressed through directives from medical or paramedical experts, and that of the administration, comprised of managers responsible for overseeing the facility's operations. However, the administration's approach to care activities differs significantly from that of clinical experts, which inevitably influences the approach to developing cognitive aids.

Hospital managers have long been importing turnkey managerial techniques from the industrial world, where management is a constantly evolving discipline (Minvielle 2018). Presently, in the healthcare domain, a prevailing representation characterizing care activity is that of process control. Building on industrial engineering principles, organizational engineering has embraced the concept of "process". Examples of processes within a hospital include medication supply, care delivery, hospital hospitality and, notably, the patient pathway, which serves as the central process underpinning the operations of a healthcare facility.

According to Georges and Samson (2012), a process in the healthcare field is defined as "a series of well-described actions, to be undertaken in order, to solve known health problems with stable results, as quickly as possible, while minimizing costs" (ibid., p. 164). Standardization should consistently yield the same results. The establishment of a care production line must ensure speed, cost minimization and efficiency through resource rationalization. Qualitative and quantitative indicators, organized in dashboards, enable the monitoring of process operations.

Similar to guidelines, the concept of standardization is evident in managerial directives. However, this standardization does not stem from the biomedical knowledge base but rather from managerial projects that need to be translated into processes that describe the expected activity within the organization. A process embodies a project's realization, representing an ideal approach for implementing the project in practice.

In a process, stakeholders can have different roles.

– Executor: staff execute the operations necessary to transform the process inputs into outputs (the patient enters ill, and exits recovered).

– Driver: some stakeholders are responsible for ensuring the proper functioning of the process. For instance, the pharmacist manages the medication circuit, the nursing manager coordinates care and the physician oversees the medical record. These drivers must describe the state of the process for which they are responsible and regularly analyze it during work meetings.

– Supplier or customer of the process: they are respectively responsible for providing inputs and ensuring outputs of the process, themselves being part of other upstream and downstream processes. Their interaction with the process raises the issue of the interface between several different processes. They must coordinate with each other to form an overall process that is efficient (Benoît and Passerat-Boulade 2020).

If the process is the focus of hospital managers' work, it implies that their scope is not directly related to patient care but rather to the operation of a facility. This distinction is important because it introduces a managerial definition of work aids that differs from that provided by clinical experts.

5.2.1. *Cognitive aids for organizational functioning*

Once the process has become the primary unit for characterizing healthcare work, cognitive aids then serve as tools to *facilitate the operation of the process*. Three main forms of action can be considered that involve cognitive aids: formalizing the process, ensuring its rational functioning and evaluating it.

– *Formalizing the process*: formalizing and elucidating a process to establish a clear delineation and representation of this aspect of a healthcare institution's activity. This task of clarification falls within the scope of managers, as well as drivers who must possess a comprehensive understanding of the sector they oversee. Various documents are available to support this formalization effort such as the process identity sheet (PIS), which offers a framework for detailing a process's characteristics, objectives, performance indicators, drivers and their authority. Within this document, each process is described using psychological instruments such as flowcharts, diagrams and tables (Benoît and Passerat-Boulade 2020).

– *Ensuring the rational functioning of the process*: hospital managerial literature specifies that a document describing a process, once drafted by an expert, can guide a non-expert while maintaining consistent quality and efficiency. Following the logic of neo-Taylorism and task automation, if the process is highly formalized and precisely described in documents, it is understood that this process can be easily standardized and delegated to potentially less qualified personnel than those involved in its initial formalization (Georges and Samson 2012). In this context, cognitive aids are seen as a means of ensuring that managerial instructions are followed by operators. From the described process emerges a working procedure that serves as guidelines to be followed. It is "a kind of regulation whose deviation is measured" (Georges and Samson 2012, p. 165).

– *Evaluating the process*: certain caregivers who hold the role of process leaders are tasked with a critical managerial function of assessing the process they oversee. To perform this task, they must gather data on performance and risks. In France, campaigns such as IPAQSS (Indicators for the Improvement of Quality and Care) serve this purpose. A central cognitive aid in this endeavor is the dashboard, designed to aggregate a range of activity indicators. These dashboards for each process within the institution are reported by the institution's management to national agencies such as HAS and ANESM.

Note that the various cognitive aids underlying these three forms of action represent an effort towards a more analytical mindset, an approach often observed when ensuring the implementation of prescribed tasks in the field.

Through this managerial approach, two forms of interrelating risks need to be considered: the risk of interference between the repository of prescribed tasks from managers and that from biomedical directives; the risk of assimilating the care activity into a technical-industrial process.

– *Interference between the two forms of prescribed tasks*: care as a process or as medical care of a patient represents two perspectives of the same domain that can collide. This is evident in the growing weight of administrative procedures on caregivers' activities (Granger 2022). Working documents often serve administrative functions rather than supporting patient care. An illustrative example of this conflict is a patient charter, presented in a hospital management book: during an upcoming organizational performance audit in an establishment, administrative services realize that the patient rights charter is not displayed in the facility. An immediate correction is made to meet the requirements of the audit firm that is to arrive soon. The author's comments on this example are of interest, as he suggests that a deeper analysis of the root causes of this oversight should have been conducted to prevent recurrence. This example illustrates how situations are interpreted based on deviations from organizational indicators (presence of a displayed charter) without considering the document's value in patient care. Indeed, if an analysis of the dysfunction is considered, its objective is to prevent this omission from recurring. No questions are raised about the intrinsic value of this document, its format or its readability. Was this document really useful and usable as it was by the users? The purpose of the document, its content, as a cognitive aid for users are not questioned. The investigation will only seek to highlight a poorly managed document management process. Another example is symbolic but equally revealing of a shift in cognitive aids towards administrative references; it concerns the surgical checklist. While the original version proposed by the WHO is limited to items to be checked, the French version proposed by the National Authority for Health has added the need for a physician's signature. In addition to supporting thinking, the surgical checklist has become a formal document involving accountability.

– *The activity of care assimilated into a technical-industrial process*: fundamentally, the risk of invoking the concept of a process is to equate the care activity with an industrial process. Naturally, it is clear that the use of this concept does not imply, in the minds of its users, that the patient is reduced to a mere product on a production line. This assimilation occurs at a more abstract level. However, even at a high level of abstraction, applying the notion of a process can have implications for the design of cognitive aids for caregivers.

However, there is not necessarily a fundamental incompatibility between viewing patient care as both a qualitative care activity and as a process integrated into a broader system of flows and resources to be managed. These two perspectives can complement each other and generate synergy. A tangible example of such complementarity, manifested within an information system, is the PsyStart system.

5.2.2. *An example of cognitive aid to care for and manage: the PsyStart system*

The PsyStart system is an information system developed in the United States for the psychological care of victims following disasters such as hurricanes, fires or industrial accidents (Schreiber 2010). Essentially, this system relies on a simple cognitive aid for rescuers: a triage sheet for victims based on criteria that assesses their risk of experiencing post-traumatic stress disorder (PTSD). To enable rescuers to assess this risk easily and concretely, without requiring in-depth knowledge of mental health, items on the PsyStart triage sheet focus primarily on describing what the victim has experienced: delayed evacuation from the disaster site, loss of a loved one, somatic injuries, loss of home, witnessing deaths, etc. The device could have stopped at this medical-psychological function, providing valuable cognitive assistance to rescuers without the necessary expertise for a rigorous psychological diagnosis. However, the system goes further by using the information collected through the triage tool to enhance the situational awareness of coordination teams managing rescue efforts. Through a shared and geolocated information system, these data that describe the experiences of victims help to estimate at a given triage location the impact of the disaster on homes and the extent of the catastrophe in a given area. These insights serve as indicators for managing the logistical deployment of rescue resources. For rescue coordination, the information from the triage sheet serves not as indicators of the victims' psychological states, but rather as guides for directing human and material resources to the affected area. In this context, cognitive aid functions as an instrument at different levels, allowing different perspectives to be extracted from the same dataset, some relevant to direct users (caregivers, rescuers), and others relevant to managers. As a result, the goals of care and management are no longer in conflict. The contributions of the PsyStart system were demonstrated by the American Red Cross during Hurricane Sandy, which devastated several states in the United States in 2012 (Schreiber et al. 2014).

Furthermore, it is worth noting that while managers can use clinical indicators to devise management metrics, the reverse is also true. For instance, indicators regarding the operation of a department or institution can serve epidemiological study purposes.

The challenge of developing work aids like PsyStart, with synergistic value, may stem from a fundamental misunderstanding about the nature of caregiving activity and, consequently, how to provide assistance. As observed, aeronautics witnessed the emergence of the first cognitive aids. This domain serves as a model not only for crafting cognitive aids in the healthcare domain but also for considering risk management strategies more broadly. However, while parallels can be drawn between aeronautics and certain medical activities, the two fields diverge significantly in certain aspects. Essentially, piloting an aircraft involves managing a technological process, aligning with the managerial concept of caregiving as part of a process. Nevertheless, flying an airplane differs fundamentally from treating a patient. On the one hand, we encounter a system with tight coupling, while, on the other hand, a system with loose coupling.

5.3. Care: a system with tight coupling

Coupling can be described as a mechanism in which two gears are more or less dependent on each other. When the coupling is tight, the operation of one gear consistently drives the operation of the other, as seen in a motor. However, when the coupling is loose, the interaction between the two gears is indirect, and the effects of one gear on the other are less predictable. This introduces uncertainty.

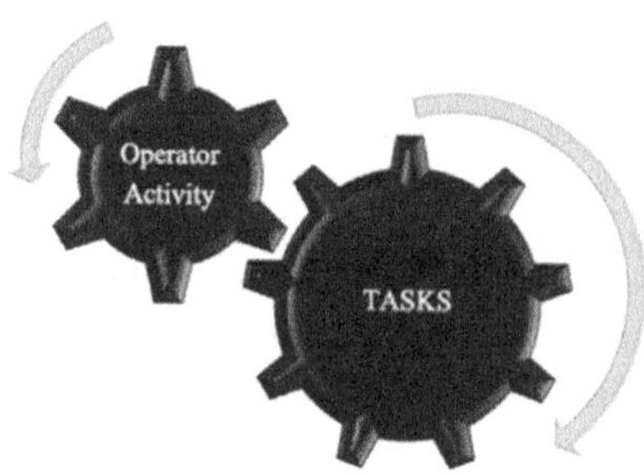

Figure 5.4. *A direct coupling between the expected tasks (directives, protocols, managerial instructions) and the actual activity of the operators*

At a workstation, coupling refers to the coordination between the tasks that operators are required to perform and their actual activity at a given moment (Figure 5.4). If the coupling is systematic, the operators' activity will fully align with the prescribed tasks (protocols), as defined to optimize the process's operation. In aircraft piloting, this mode of operation is common, although ergonomics has shown that there are always more or less significant discrepancies between what is prescribed and what is achieved. In the field of caregiving, a high coupling corresponds to type A strategies in René Amalberti's nomenclature, accounting for 40% of cases according to the author. In reality, caregiving exhibits a set of characteristics that make it a working system with relatively loose coupling compared to technical-industrial systems.

5.3.1. *A coupling to be developed*

During their work at any given moment, an airplane pilot has objectives and an operational procedure to achieve those objectives. In the field of healthcare, the "caregiver–patient" relationship is not as well defined in terms of future tasks from the outset of the interaction. Faced with a new patient, uncertainty prevails regarding the nature of the pathology and the medical or paramedical tasks that will result from it. The caregiver's activity will therefore involve seeking to understand the patient's condition (diagnosis) in order to plan a care regimen to restore them to a "normal" state, normatively referred to as "health", but which remains fundamentally vague. The outcome of the diagnosis is crucial. It is through this that the mental representation formed by the caregiver can correspond to the reality of the patient's condition, initiating a functional coupling with a care plan to follow. This care plan will be developed primarily by the caregiver, but the patient or family may also contribute to it to some extent. In other words, future tasks are chosen based on the situation, and the coupling to be achieved with goals to be attained is constructed simultaneously.

In a technical-industrial domain such as aeronautics, the issue of establishing coupling is far less central to the activity. It is highly probable that the technical device, the aircraft, operates nominally, and pilots do not need to exert any particular effort to "understand" the state of an aircraft, which itself does not have a perspective to communicate to the pilots. Coupling occurs from the outset. It is only in situations of malfunction that a diagnostic activity must be undertaken to understand what is happening and restore the device to normal operation. However, in clinical practice, caregivers are not consistently engaged in problem-solving when encountering a new patient. Leveraging clinical knowledge, they use expertise to identify stable patterns in the symptoms a person presents, facilitating the development of automated reasoning processes. Nevertheless, fundamentally, the initiation of coupling between the patient and the caregiver is not immediately established. For instance, a physician greeting a patient in consultation would not ask "How are you?" (the context implicitly suggests a negative response), but rather "What brings you here?" (implying a health-related issue). Yet, before takeoff, if we were to accept the notion of the pilot conversing with the aircraft, their initial checks could be akin to asking "How are you?". The beginning of the interaction is not of the same nature, leading to a different perspective on, for example, a verification checklist in the medical field compared to one in aeronautics.

5.3.2. *A nonlinear and uncertain causal relationship*

When the coupling is tight between tasks and real activity, every action of the operators in the workspace generates a predictable effect on the domain. In the cockpit, an action on a control produces a direct effect that can be easily anticipated. This is the "push-button" effect. Conversely, an event affecting the aircraft's dynamics, such as encountering turbulence, will have foreseeable consequences on piloting. This high certainty about cause-and-effect relationships theoretically allows for the replacement of pilots with automatons. This is evident with the existence of autopilots or automatic drones capable of tracking a target without any human intervention. When the coupling is loose, this linear causality between actions and effects on the domain is no longer present. The effect of a medical procedure or therapy on a patient retains a considerable degree of uncertainty regarding the outcomes it will produce, and the effects may not be immediately observable. They often take a nonlinear form with threshold effects. To paraphrase the Swiss physician and alchemist Paracelsus (1493–1541): "Everything is poison, nothing is poison, only the dose makes the poison". The laws of physiology and medicine do not exhibit the same linearity and predictability as the laws of physics and the kinematics of flying vehicles.

The loose coupling within healthcare systems undermines the possibility of a simple, direct and certain effect of instructions and protocol follow-ups, as well as a simple, direct and certain effect of cognitive aids on care. In a system with high coupling, cognitive aids (checklists, decision aids, to-do lists, etc.) are direct vectors of prescriptions used to drive the functioning of the system's gears. The information contained in the cognitive aid "travels" through the operators and their activity, and then the domain is modified accordingly. Checklists, manuals used by pilots activate the system to operate in accordance with the expected prescribed tasks. *In systems with loose coupling like those in the healthcare field, the role of a direct gateway between task and activity that cognitive aids could have is not immediately ensured.* While a technical device to be piloted can be termed complicated due to the technology underlying it, a living organism to be treated can be termed complex due to its uncertainty, high variability, and the multiple resulting interactions.

5.3.3. *A workspace characterized by high variability*

The high variability of work configurations in the healthcare field makes achieving a high level of coupling difficult. First, patient profiles are diverse, and the condition of the same patient evolves over time. Additionally, caregivers often attend to multiple patients simultaneously. This aspect has a significant consequence: simultaneously managing several patients creates a unique work configuration within a given time interval, different from previous ones. On the team side, their composition frequently changes, preventing the establishment of a stable common mode of operation based on routines. This variability in team composition reduces the opportunities to develop shared knowledge patterns and work habits. Shared operating procedures have the advantage of reducing the need for explicit exchanges between teammates by creating implicit expectation frameworks. In a cockpit, even if the pilot and copilot do not know each other, they have some time to get acquainted before takeoff, and furthermore, they ultimately form a pair, the smallest team possible. Operating procedures are so standardized that they inherently share implicit expectation frameworks.

In the face of these various uncertainties in caregiving, a range of work strategies is necessary to deal with a variety of different situations. This central idea is articulated in a principle put forth by cyberneticist[1] Ross Ashby. It is known as the *law of requisite variety* (Ashby 1958; Hollnagel 2011). Ashby explains this principle using the analogy of a living organism confronted with an environment populated by potentially hostile bacteria. For this organism to have the best chance of survival, it must have a variety of "friendly" bacteria in its internal biotope as wide as the variety of "enemy" bacteria outside capable of attacking it. Applied to a work system, this means that *in the face of a domain presenting a variety of demands, the organization must have a range of strategies as broad as possible to respond to these demands appropriately*. In this context, the variability of observable operating modes among caregivers is not a flaw that should be systematically trimmed, homogenized or standardized, as tends to be suggested by process management logic. On the contrary, this multiplicity allows teams to have a repertoire of responses to deal with the diversity of work configurations they encounter (Flach 2012).

The law of requisite variety operationally explains the notion of resilience. Resilience corresponds to the capacity to confront a situation regardless of its nature or the magnitude of constraints and difficulties it presents. *If certain work systems, such as healthcare systems, exhibit loose coupling, it is because the need for resilience dominates in their interaction with the work domain*. This objective may even supersede that of performance, which remains a primary criterion in highly coupled systems like aeronautics. Confronted with the diverse work configurations in the hospital environment and the pressures exerted by these configurations on personnel, resilience must be prioritized before seeking to optimize a standardized mode of operation. To embody resilience, a healthcare system uses various strategies.

1 Cybernetics is the science of self-regulating systems.

5.3.4. *Resilience provided by loose coupling*

Preventing a healthcare system from operating as fully interdependent gears allows for degrees of freedom to deal with unexpected events. This involves introducing some flexibility, also known as "slack", between the gears, so as not to generate a predefined and direct response to every demand, as tasks are often defined within a process-driven logic (Basso Verle et al. 2019). Such a work configuration will inevitably impact the definition of the role of cognitive aid.

Consider the example of exceptional healthcare situations, which demand significant adaptation to the unexpected. Institutionally, internal hospital mobilization plans and the "Plan Blanc" or white plans in France represent typical organizational responses to handle degraded situations (such as influxes of casualties, epidemics, nuclear, radiological or chemical accidents, degraded functioning of facilities, infections affecting services, alteration of care provision) (Ministère des Solidarités et de la Santé 2019). However, these plans constitute prescribed tasks rather than a description of real activity. In disaster contexts, adhering strictly to these prescriptions can be particularly challenging. Moreover, the macroscopic description of strategies for these exceptional situations does not reflect the resilience strategies that emerge at the team or workstation level, observable even in daily scenarios when various constraints unexpectedly increase (Morineau and Flach 2019). In these contexts, resilience strategies concerning patient reception, care or referral are implemented. This resilience often leads to the creation of support mechanisms to address the increased constraints of a degraded situation. Below are some strategies:

– *Improvisation and innovation*: the diversity of work contexts and the emergence of degraded situations in emergencies make the medical field, and more generally, emergency services a sector in which improvisation is likely to emerge as a resilience strategy. Mendonça and Wallace (2007) propose a two-step model to describe improvisation: in step 1, recognizing that no predefined plan is available, or that a predefined plan would be suitable but cannot be implemented due to a lack of necessary resources; in step 2, conceptualizing and executing a novel plan.

Improvisation allows for ad hoc adaptation, grounded in *creativity*, which involves proposing new alternatives to achieve an objective. Drawing from field observations, document collection, reports, maps and journalistic articles, Kendra and Wachtendorf (2003) examined the creativity demonstrated by various rescue services during the September 11, 2001, World Trade Center attack. During this disaster, between 500,000 and 1 million people were evacuated from Manhattan by tourist boats, military ships, ferries or private boats. As the New York Rescue Coordination Center was situated at 7 World Trade Center, it had to be relocated first to a truck, then to the Port of New York. Rescuers, and even ordinary New

Yorkers displayed creativity in their efforts to contribute to the relief operation. Examples include bicycle couriers delivering food along the secure zone and physiotherapists supporting coordination teams by providing care on carpets laid on top of stacks of pallets.

Improvisation is typically a temporary strategy, which is used to address the unusual constraints of an activity. If the operational approach stabilizes over time and becomes shared, it can lead to genuine innovations. During the Covid-19 crisis, numerous improvisations emerged to cope with this unprecedented situation, often resulting in significant innovations. For instance, in Italy, at the onset of the Covid-19 pandemic, doctors ingeniously repurposed the EasyBreath (Decathlon) diving mask to serve as an oxygenation mask. This adaptation was subsequently validated by an international team and distributed in many countries. It is worth noting that improvisation in emergency scenarios frequently spawns *frugal innovation*, driven by resource scarcity and the urgent need for equipment or methodologies. Frugal innovation involves a DIY approach. Furthermore, it is noteworthy that technological innovations in the incubation phase experienced sudden acceleration during the pandemic. For instance, telemedicine and telecommuting, which were in nascent stages prior to the Covid-19 crisis, rapidly evolved to become integrated into mainstream practices across numerous organizations.

– *Reprioritization of activities*: reprioritizing the reception, care or referral of a set of patients is a means to address a new work configuration, such as an influx of victims after a disaster. To achieve this capability, it is necessary to step beyond the framework established by the instructions typically applied, and to alter the triage and decision-making criteria. At the onset and peak of the Covid-19 pandemic in Italy, 10–25% of hospitalized patients because of the virus required artificial respiration, while the number of ventilators was insufficient. Doctors had to conduct triages under the pressure of new criteria, leading to discontinuing respiratory assistance for one patient to benefit another. These novel situations of reprioritization prompted some doctors to propose a new operational mode by establishing triage committees in hospitals. The objective was to alleviate the individual pressure that such decisions placed on doctors, who often found themselves alone in making them (Truog et al. 2020). These committees comprised volunteer practitioners and experts who were not directly involved in the care of the affected patients. However, caregivers directly involved could appeal a decision made by the committee.

– *Resource reorganization*: when faced with malfunctions or shortages of human or material resources, teams must be capable of reorganizing their operational methods, stepping out of the predefined roles and sometimes changing material means, including using alternative devices. The Covid-19 health crisis demonstrated the resilience of teams in adapting to this new situation. For instance, the SafeTeam website describes a scenario at the onset of the pandemic, in which the first Covid-19 patient arrived at an intensive care unit. Remarkably, it was a nursing assistant who assumed leadership in organizing the care, rather than one of the attending physicians. This nursing assistant had prior experience in receiving Covid-19 patients, enabling her to guide the management based on her firsthand experience (SafeTeam 2020). Additionally, regarding material resources, the transition to "paper" operations following a cyber-attack, such as the one witnessed in September 2022 at the Corbeilles-Essonne hospital, which rendered digital terminals inoperative, necessitated a restructuring of work processes. These adaptations underscore the importance of applying the law of requisite variety by leveraging alternative resources that may lie dormant within the teams, whether in the form of untapped skills (like the leadership of a caregiver) or neglected materials, such as paper-based documentation.

– *Redundancy*: in the pursuit of performance optimization, redundancy involves the repetition of an activity, thus slowing down the treatment process. Within a managerial model centered on streamlined operational processes, redundancy may be perceived as a waste of time and resources. However, in the context of resilience, redundancy serves to enhance the reliability of activities that may otherwise be compromised by situational constraints. For instance, in emergency scenarios, requiring patients to provide their name multiple times may prolong overall patient management. Nonetheless, this practice helps to prevent critical errors with a high likelihood of occurrence.

– *Implementation of "shock absorbers"*: in the context of process logic, an individual (such as a patient), an object (e.g. medication) or information should ideally move through the process in which they are involved as swiftly as possible. This principle places the process under strain, meaning it operates at maximum capacity continuously, especially when inputs remain relatively constant. Such conditions make it challenging to incorporate additional activities, such as handling a new event alongside regular operations. Consequently, the process loses its flexibility and ability to adapt to the unexpected. To borrow the terminology of Cook and Rasmussen (2005), the process becomes "solid".

Various types of elements can interfere in the main activity. This may include additional tasks, such as checkpoints facilitated by checklists, debriefings, on-the-job training for internship students or support for internal students. Unplanned events can disrupt the process, such as a sudden influx of patients, technical malfunctions or insufficient resources to work. In response to these risks, it is essential to establish *shock absorbers* within the activity. *These "shock absorbers" delay the activity in comparison to what would be expected optimally, preferably before the occurrence of an unexpected event.* The goal is to preserve degrees of freedom that make it possible to absorb the impact of increased activity, events endangering the system's operation or enhance the activity's reliability by implementing a type of "freeze frame" (see Figure 5.5).

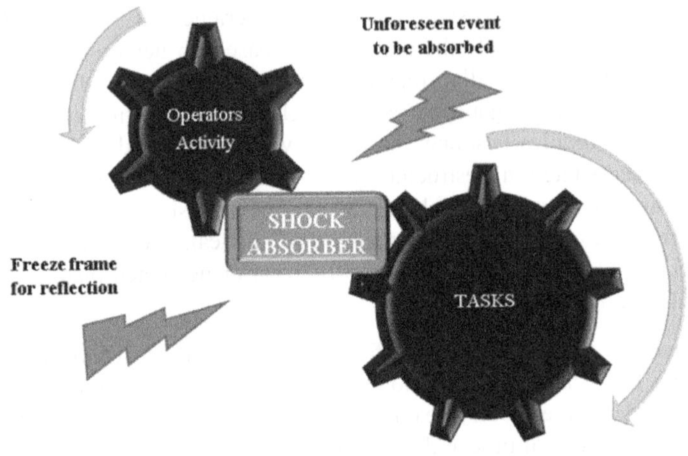

Figure 5.5. *Operation of a loosely coupled system equipped with shock absorbers to address an unforeseen event or to allow for moments of reflection*

Various forms of shock absorbers can be identified.

– *Spatial shock absorbers*: an example of a spatial shock absorber is management of beds in a resuscitation department. The need to accommodate a critically ill patient at any time requires that bed occupancy in the ward not be continuously overloaded. This involves being prepared to receive a victim for whom care would be highly critical (Basso Werle et al. 2019).

– *Temporal shock absorbers*: in an emergency department, the act of waiting for a patient at a given moment can be intentionally caused by the doctor who places the patient in an observation phase, essential for monitoring the evolution of their condition. "Act then wait to see" is a fundamental heuristic in medical care (Mol 2008). Arbitrarily reducing the time between entries and exits in a service may ultimately diminish the quality of care.

– *Buffers*: shock absorbers can also pertain to information storage. These are referred to as *buffers*, which are external memory spaces transiently storing information between two processing steps. The implementation of verification moments in the activity falls under this type of shock absorber. For instance, the operating room checklist creates buffers by introducing three interludes between the induction of anesthesia, surgery and the patient's departure from the operating room, in addition to the high coupling it seeks to achieve by explicating the *items to be checked*.

Instead of merely acting as intermediaries to enhance the coupling between tasks and actual activities, certain cognitive aids for a loosely coupled system can primarily contribute to the creation of spatial, temporal or informational shock absorbers.

An example of such a practice is the implementation of briefing moments within the operations of a healthcare service. During a work analysis conducted in an emergency department, it was noted that physicians and paramedical staff situated in two different offices encountered challenges in exchanging patient information. With the support of the teams and a working group, a concept termed "coordination points" was tested. At three pre-defined times (midnight, 8:30 a.m. and 3:30 p.m.), all staff members in the department were required to gather in front of a large screen displaying the current patients, facilitating discussions on medical records and fostering a comprehensive awareness of the situation. Initially, during the trial phase, some staff members expressed concerns about feeling as though they were wasting time or experiencing decreased efficiency by engaging in these "freeze frame" moments. However, two years later, the practice remained in place and became an integral part of the staff's routine. An anonymous online survey conducted with the teams revealed that the majority of respondents believed that coordination points improved information sharing within the team: 78% fully agreed with this observation, while 20% agreed (46 respondents). Particularly noteworthy was the perception that coordination points helped to prevent certain patients being overlooked, with 72% fully agreeing and 17% agreeing with this assertion (47 respondents). Therefore, the perceived time loss associated with these meeting points ultimately translates into enhanced operational efficiency and resilience for the service (Morineau and Djenidi-Delfour 2023).

All of these resilient strategies typically involve the collective workforce, which redefines operational methods on-site. The collective itself serves as an essential form of cognitive support to address sudden constraints, which are challenging for isolated individuals to deal with, let alone the emotional support provided by the collective workforce when facing the psychological burden brought about by certain situations involving suffering or death. In these contexts, each individual within the group acts as a bridge to others, providing support to sustain work activities.

5.3.5. *Risks of considering care as tight coupling: the case of alarms*

Alarms represent a cognitive aid that typically embodies an approach to a work system from the perspective of tight coupling. An event or action directly triggers an alarm. Subsequently, operators are tasked with promptly responding to the alarm, with the initial response being to validate it by pressing a button to deactivate it. However, the ECRI institute, an American organization studying healthcare systems, highlighted in 2012 that alarm technology poses the highest risk in the medical field. These risks specifically involve inappropriate changes in alarm operation, staff fatigue due to the high frequency of alarms and desensitization to their activation. Studies suggest that false alarms or alarms that lack significance (false affordances) may account for 80–99% of occurrences (Cvach 2012)! Physiological monitor alarms are designed to be highly sensitive to any variations in a patient's vital signs to avoid overlooking changes in their condition. While this sensitivity in trigger thresholds reflects the engineers' commendable intention, it simultaneously increases the likelihood of false alarms. Alarms then become a nuisance in themselves. They no longer induce reactions. Healthcare providers ignore them or deactivate them (risk of hidden affordance). On the contrary, alarm designers accustomed to operating in stable "dashboard" environments design sensors intended to be fixed. For example, monitoring alarms are designed for a patient lying down, not moving, which is often not the case. As a result, many false alarms are related to patient movements producing artifacts.

Instead of adhering to fixed trigger thresholds, Cvach (2012) suggests adjusting the thresholds based on the patient's profile and documenting them in the medical record. This approach should also consider the acoustic environment of the surroundings. Engineering efforts are aimed at developing "smart alarms" capable of automatically adapting to the triggering contexts. Such comprehensive consideration of alarms arises from recognizing the variability of healthcare situations, thereby acknowledging the need to view them as loosely coupled. It places the crucial dimension of patient state monitoring at the forefront of care, a dimension often relegated to a peripheral role in caregivers' activities, as they have become accustomed to adapting to alarm failures and opting to "deal with it". In contrast, in aviation, such alarm malfunctions would be deemed unacceptable and promptly addressed. However, addressing alarm issues in a loosely coupled work system is far more intricate than adjusting trigger thresholds in an aircraft cockpit. Alarms serve as challenging cognitive aids to implement in a fluctuating and dynamic environment, where multiple events and contexts disrupt sensor operation and the qualitative interpretation of displayed values. Nevertheless, these physiological sensors are indispensable for monitoring a patient's condition. An alternative approach involves developing cognitive aids tailored to loosely coupled work systems.

Previously, we discussed coordination points as an example of cognitive aid implemented to facilitate the operation of a healthcare service within a framework of loose coupling. Another example of cognitive aid designed to support this specific logic in healthcare is an admission form used in an emergency department.

5.3.6. *An example of aid for loose coupling: the welcome sheet in emergency rooms*

A hospital process under particularly high pressure is patient reception in the emergency room. The almost continuous influx of visitors generates a heavy workload, especially for triage nurses who are responsible for conducting initial clinical assessments, prioritizing patients based on the severity of their condition and directing them to the appropriate medical zone. Within the framework of the process, triage nurses, like other emergency healthcare providers, are tasked with streamlining the patient's journey to minimize waiting times and congestion, which could adversely affect critically ill patients (a concept of tight coupling). However, fluidity should not be equated with haste, as this could lead to unintended consequences. To cope with the pressure resulting from patient admissions, triage nurses require support to moderate the pace, ensure reliable reception and adapt to ad hoc work reorganizations. In essence, they need the means to implement resilience strategies.

5.3.6.1. *Highly interrupted reception work*

During the summer holidays, observing the work of triage nurses at the emergency department of the Bretagne Atlantique Hospital Center in Vannes (a tourist city) helped to make clear the constraints of their activity and thus design a cognitive aid to support the information processing of triage nurses (Morineau et al. 2021). During the daytime observation period, an average of 227 visits per 24 hours was recorded. While creating 34 patient files, triage nurses experienced an average of one task interruption every minute (0.9 interruptions more precisely). These interruptions contribute to mental load and stress, as they require triage nurses to hold information in memory while switching tasks, increasing the risk of omissions, redundancies in information retrieval and errors in data integration into patient files.

5.3.6.2. *Creation of a "buffer": the "1st contact" sheet*

To cope with these constraints, a paper sheet was designed in collaboration with the teams and as part of a working group within the department (Figure 5.6).

This compact sheet (A5 size) is assembled as a bundle of detachable pages, easily storable in a gown pocket, yet allowing for effortless writing in the palm of the hand, as the bundle serves as a physical support. In this regard, it offers a range of affordances, tangible features that facilitate its use by nurses who need to move between workstations and patients. Its content covers essential information to be gathered and allows for annotations to address varying situations (resilience). The purpose of this sheet is to serve as a buffer, temporarily storing information about a patient upon arrival at the reception. In essence, this sheet is designed to:

– delay information processing: enabling a “freeze frame” regarding a patient to address other priority requests promptly;

– collect highly variable information: facilitating improvisation in gathering patient-specific details;

– be disposable after use: serving as temporary memory storage with transient usefulness, without imposing additional document management tasks;

– be usable at the healthcare provider’s discretion without strict obligation: providing an extra level of flexibility in information gathering, rather than a mandated constraint. The triage nurse may opt for alternative strategies, such as using their own short-term memory for temporary information storage.

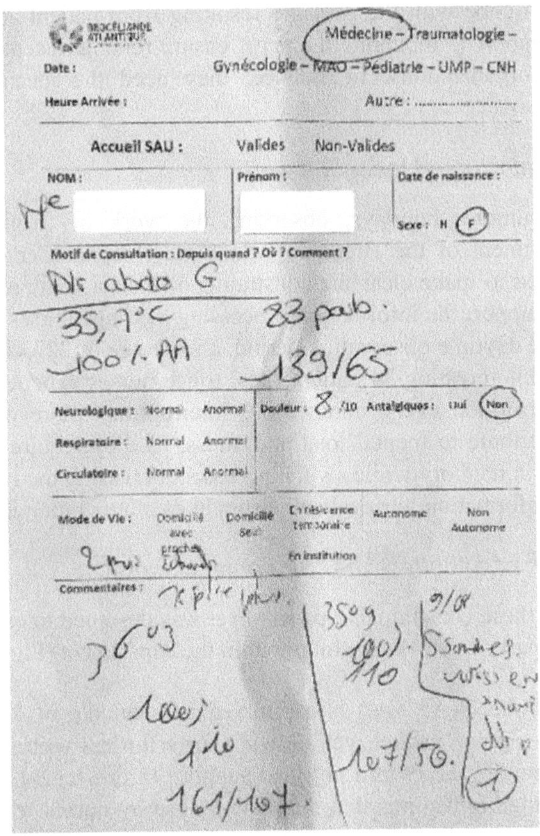

Médecine – Traumatologie – Gynécologie – MAO – Pédiatrie – UMP – CNH

Date :

Heure Arrivée :

Autre :

Accueil SAU : Valides Non-Valides

NOM : | Prénom : | Date de naissance :

Sexe : H F

Motif de Consultation : Depuis quand ? Où ? Comment ?

Neurologique : Normal Anormal | Douleur : /10 Antalgiques : Oui Non

Respiratoire : Normal Anormal

Circulatoire : Normal Anormal

Mode de Vie : Domicilié avec proches | Domicilié Seul | Convalescence temporaire | Autonome | Non Autonome | En institution

Commentaires :

Figure 5.6. *Example of a “1st contact” sheet used during the activity (Morineau et al. (2021), Bretagne Atlantique Hospital Center). For a color version of this figure, see www.iste.co.uk/morineau/cognitive.zip*

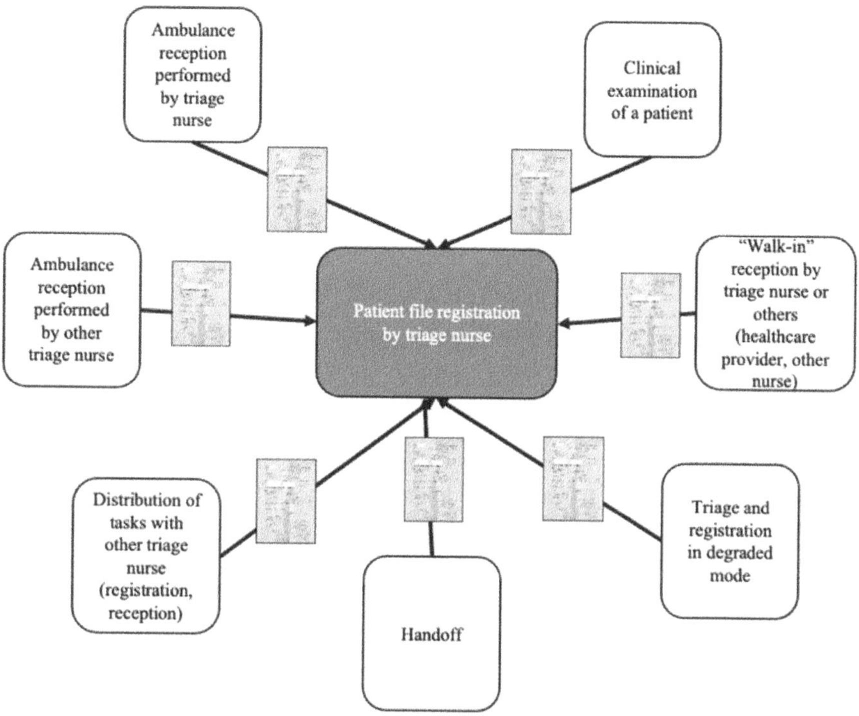

Figure 5.7. *The buffer functions of the "1st contact" sheet between patient registration tasks and other tasks*

5.3.6.3. *Results of implementing the "1st contact" sheet*

Observation of the use of the sheet, along with an anonymously distributed online questionnaire 10 months after its implementation, highlights its role as a genuine support for resilience. The document serves as a buffer, allowing the triage nurse to free up short-term memory when transitioning from one task to another (Figure 5.7). It enables quick storage of information about the patient transported on a stretcher, thus allowing firefighters or ambulance personnel to be released promptly. Sometimes, it is used as a tool to note the evolution of the patient's physiological parameters. The example sheet presented in Figure 5.6 illustrates this additional function, which was not originally specified in the design. The sheet also facilitates information exchange within the team. Typically, walk-in reception is handled by a triage nurse, but in cases of work overload, a nursing assistant may perform this task. The sheet helps to distribute patient care among triage nurses when they work in pairs, based on their assigned positions and workload. It also serves as a tool during shift handovers.

Finally, practice has revealed that it could serve as an alternative means to address a degraded situation. This was evident during a two-hour period when the computer system used at the reception was offline. The sheet then functioned as a fallback for triaging and registering patients. Survey results indicate that 7 out of 10 participants oppose reverting to the previous operation, namely, without the presence of the sheet.

This cognitive aid was conceived not to heighten the level of coupling between patient arrivals and the caregivers' activities, but rather as a means to "*add flexibility*" *to the system, thereby opening up degrees of freedom to create opportunities for managing the numerous constraints that operators face simultaneously and addressing situations of work overload where coupling needs to be loose.* However, in the healthcare domain, the activities surrounding care are diverse. Each medical or paramedical specialty presents specific constraints that categorize it as either loosely or tightly coupled. Consequently, the analogy with the aviation domain (tight coupling) may vary in its applicability depending on the specialty.

5.3.7. *Coupling nuances in the health field*

A specific yet common medical scenario involves the patient being under anesthesia. In such a setting, the patient is surrounded by technical apparatus ensuring the essential physiological functions for survival and monitoring, as seen during anesthesia in the operating room or in an intensive care unit. The workflow system in these cases is notably tightly coupled. This is why the field of anesthesia has often been likened to airplane piloting, as noted in the works of anesthesiologist Gaba in the United States. Certain aspects of anesthesia, such as the phases of induction and emergence, resemble the takeoff and landing of an aircraft. During these phases, like airplane pilots, the anesthesiologist and nurse anesthetist (the "pilot" and "co-pilot") must monitor various variables on a monitor to ensure the smooth progression of patient care. Similarly, on the surgical side, procedures are characterized by a relatively high level of coupling. Evidence of this lies in the surgeon's ability to anticipate the course of a surgical procedure quite precisely, often even before its commencement, based solely on observations of medical imaging of the operative area (Morineau et al. 2009a).

Emergency medicine, however, is arguably the medical field with one of the loosest couplings between patients and care teams. By its very nature, emergencies involve high levels of variability and uncertainty. However, when we delve into the various types of emergency care, we can refine the measurement of coupling degrees. In a resuscitation bay for managing critical emergencies, once a diagnosis is established, the care protocol is often highly standardized, with predefined actions, assigned roles, timeframes to be adhered to and multiple sensors monitoring the patient. Conversely, emergency care in out-of-hospital contexts, especially in extreme environments such as conflict zones or amid natural disasters, demands improvisation and on-the-spot adaptations based on site configurations and victim numbers. Sometimes, due to limited resources, equipment may be repurposed, such as using a belt as a tourniquet or makeshift stretchers made from metal barriers, as observed during the evacuation of Bataclan victims (Langlois and Ploquin 2016). Therefore, the analogy between aeronautics and medical care varies depending on medical specialties. It is crucial to finely analyze the coupling degree within a workstation or department to guide the functions that the cognitive aid should have, whether focused on performance or resilience.

5.4. Conclusion

Understanding cognitive aids as gateways between prescribed tasks and real-world activity reminds us that the cognitive system comprising caregivers and their work environment is a functional system directed by goals to be achieved and applied in context. One of the unique aspects of cognitive systems in the healthcare field is that they are driven by two forms of goals: those set by domain experts and those set by hospital managers responsible for the actual functioning of the institution. These goal forms are developed based on significantly different representations of care, which can lead to conflicts or overemphasis on one representation over another, such as when administrative document processing overrides clinical activity. Moreover, the effectiveness of clinical guidelines issued by expert committees may be diminished if they are difficult to implement in practice. To be operational, these guidelines must be reformulated into various forms of cognitive aids tailored to the activity contexts. The more constrained the work context is by the number of actions and temporal pressure, the more essential it becomes to translate directives into cognitive aids that effectively filter crucial information for presentation. These aids should be easily accessible and ergonomic to facilitate quick comprehension. Lastly, the example of the PsyStart rescue system demonstrates *the feasibility of designing "Swiss army knife" cognitive aids, providing data useful to both caregivers and managers without interfering with each other's activities.*

Another critical point affecting cognitive aids in their role as intermediaries between prescribed tasks and real-world activity is the representation used by the prescribers to characterize the care activity. On the managerial side, the metaphor of process steering conveys the idea that care activity operates like tightly coupled gears. On the domain experts' side, the metaphor of airplane piloting with the dissemination of aviation checklists in the medical world leads, through another path, to the same conclusion. In both cases, care activity is considered to be based on tight coupling between caregivers and patients. However, loose coupling is a source of resilience. It allows for the deployment of strategies to cope with the high variability of situations, even though nuances must exist depending on professional sectors, especially if caregivers work on a sedated patient for whom sensors and effectors act as technical interfaces, or they intervene in contexts with high uncertainty. *Since loose coupling in certain care situations is a source of resilience, this requires us to no longer think of cognitive aids as ways to systematically strengthen the link between real activity and expected tasks, but rather as a means to reinforce resilience strategies, for example, by implementing a buffer.*

In conclusion, and to summarize this first part of the book, considering a cognitive aid as a gateway involves defining the following:

– *Knowledge distribution between individual and environment*: it is crucial to establish a dynamic balance between what external tools provide and what should remain within the realm of internal mental operations. The real value of external aids lies in their proper use, enhancing users' internal capabilities by making them actively engaged. Externalizing knowledge should not result in passive archiving, leading to forgetfulness or skill loss.

– *Routing of knowledge from analytical or intuitive thinking*: designing a cognitive gateway prompts us to ponder the nature of knowledge and reasoning involved in daily decision-making. Are decisions based on intuition, which is challenging to verbalize, or on inferences and calculations that caregivers can readily articulate? Can routine knowledge patterns be replaced by well-formulated algorithms, or complex reasoning be transformed into easily accessible and memorizable sequences for long-term use?

– *Degree of routing requirements from instructions and directives*: crafting a cognitive gateway also involves examining the nature of the work situation and, more specifically, the relationship between operators (caregivers) and their tasks. This relationship, whether tightly or loosely coupled, allows for two possibilities: providing *assistance for performance*, ensuring strict adherence to predefined plans or *assistance for resilience*, offering freedom and "freeze frame" moments for reflection and potential modification of activities.

In all three aspects, for a cognitive gateway to be functional, it must be both easily accessible, sufficiently robust to avoid failure (reliability) and ultimately trustworthy in its ability to access the intended function, both in terms of hardware support and the informational content that the gateway routes. This conceptualization of the gateway and these criteria provide us with initial elements for the design of a cognitive aid. However, they alone are inadequate to support a comprehensive design process. Here, the metaphor of the gateway appears to reach its limits. To refine the design process, it is necessary to transition from the metaphorical language that has aided in understanding the purposes of assistive devices in order to adopt a functional model. In other words, considering cognitive aid for what it fundamentally and concretely is – an information system.

PART 2

Cognitive Aid as a Turing Machine

Introduction to Part 2

Figure I2.1. *A Turing machine, which simplistically delineates the process of reading and writing symbols executed by an entity equipped with a tape and a pencil eraser. Through this apparatus, said entity is capable of adhering to a prescribed set of instructions (state network), thereby facilitating the execution of symbol-manipulating operations*

An ergonomically designed cognitive aid, tailored to meet the requirements of its users, may be deemed as *relevant*. In terms of both informational content, physical structure and method of use, the cognitive aid should align with the characteristics of the cognitive system into which it is integrated; these characteristics encompass the demands of the working environment, the profiles of the operators and the objectives that the system aims to accomplish. Therefore, prior to delving into cognitive aids within the realm of Turing machine-type information processing systems, it is beneficial to revisit the theory of relevance in cognitive linguistics, which offers a precise definition of this concept.

Designing a relevant psychological instrument

Sperber and Wilson (1989) demonstrated in Chapter 3 that the relevance of a message incorporates both its implicit and explicit components. Another facet of their relevance theory pertains to the contextual effects and cognitive effort involved in comprehending a message.

The theory of relevance posits that in a communication scenario, *a relevant message is one that elicits maximum contextual effect in the receiver while requiring minimal cognitive effort*. The contextual effect refers to the impact of new information in relation to the receiver's existing knowledge. The greater the novelty of the transmitted information, the more it triggers a sense of surprise in the receiver, thereby generating a *contextual effect*. This notion closely aligns with Shannon's concept of information quantity in his information theory. According to Shannon, *the more improbable the content of a message ("I encountered a Martian this morning upon arriving at work"), the higher its informational content for the receiver*.

However, for a message to be processed and assimilated within a reasonable timeframe, it is imperative to consider the *cognitive effort* it demands of the receiver. To understand a message, the receiver must find a mental context, which incurs a cost. For a message to be easily understood, Sperber and Wilson propose that this cognitive cost be implicitly understood by both the sender and receiver and thus that communication be governed by a standard of relevance. It is thus tacitly agreed upon that the receiver will typically seek the least expensive cognitive context while maximizing contextual effects to interpret a new message. For example, if a colleague mentions encountering a Martian in the morning, it is preferable to interpret this remark within a humorous context, imagining the Martian as a quirky coworker rather than entertaining the costly implication of encountering an individual from Mars.

As cognitive aids serve as means of written or oral communication, it is logical to apply the standard of relevance to them. We suggest that *transposing the standard of relevance to a cognitive aid involves ensuring that its content offers information that is new to the user at a given moment, meaning information to which the user does not currently have access in order to provide assistance, while also avoiding interpretations of this information that involve excessive cognitive processing*. This principle aligns with an ideal cognitive aid.

However, while the relevance of a message in spontaneous communication is developed through ongoing interactions between two interlocutors, this standard must rely on stable criteria for cognitive assistance. Indeed, a cognitive aid is a document, or refers to a document in the case of a verbal protocol, that maintains permanence over time and remains unchanged regardless of users and situations. This necessitates translating the concepts of contextual effect and cognitive effort into criteria applicable to the content of a document.

– *Contextual effect and information completeness*: a reliable method to induce a contextual effect among a group of potential users of a cognitive aid, across various scenarios, is to furnish them with maximum information pertaining to the document's addressed domain. Conveying the comprehensive content of a care protocol or all the instructions to be adhered to should, in principle, ensure that any user discovers elements of informational support, irrespective of their expertise level or the nature of the problem they need to resolve. This approach elucidates the commonly observed inclination to devise cognitive aids aimed at delivering comprehensive information. Proceeding in this manner through *exhaustiveness* provides reassurance to the designer, ensuring that all possible scenarios have been documented.

– *Reduced cognitive effort and information selectivity*: in contrast to exhaustiveness, a reliable method to decrease cognitive effort in the user of a cognitive aid is to provide them with minimal information to process, supporting their ongoing activity. As previously discussed, this involves translating directives into specific cognitive aids, presenting a selection of content in a condensed form, similar to a reader's digest. Considering the user profile and the situation at hand, a subset of guidelines or instructions will be displayed. This prevents information overload and confusion as the user's cognitive burden in accessing the content is reduced to the maximum through this *selectivity* in the presentation of information.

– *Relevance = balance between exhaustiveness and selectivity*: the challenge in designing the content of a cognitive aid lies in satisfying these two opposing criteria – ensuring that all necessary information is communicated while also ensuring that this information is sufficient. Therefore, we encounter the equation that defines the concept of relevance as a compromise between maximizing contextual effect (exhaustiveness) and minimizing cognitive effort (selectivity).

If we return to the cognitive gateway functions outlined in Part 1 of this book to describe cognitive aids, it becomes evident that the decisions regarding the methods of transferring knowledge from one point to another, via a gateway, also involve considerations of information weighting in terms of exhaustiveness and selectivity. Table I2.1 illustrates these considerations based on whether a cognitive aid is perceived as a gateway between the individual and the environment, between intuitive and analytical thought or between prescribed tasks (directives, instructions) and actual activity.

One method to ensure exhaustiveness in the provided information is to consolidate the knowledge carried by the cognitive aid almost entirely in an external memory or in that of the operator. This occurs, for instance, when the operator memorizes a transmission protocol in a mnemonic format, or when AI software autonomously conducts all the steps of a diagnosis up to the final decision. This exhaustiveness is further guaranteed by fully explicating the knowledge and by expecting a precise and systematic follow-up of this knowledge in real-world activity.

	Exhaustiveness	Selectivity
Gateway between the individual and the environment	Knowledge consolidated in internal or external memory	Knowledge distributed within the "individual–environment" cognitive system
Gateway between intuitive and analytical thought	Maximum elaboration of knowledge (system 2 based on analysis)	Partially implicit knowledge (system 1 based on intuition)
Gateway between prescribed tasks and actual activity	Tight coupling between knowledge described in tasks and those used in actual activity	Loose coupling between knowledge described in tasks and those used in actual activity

Table I2.1. *Gateways and design choices for rather exhaustive or selective information in cognitive aid*

Conversely, a strategy to prioritize information selectivity is to distribute this information within the cognitive system among various elements of the environment and the operator. Selectivity also involves relying on implicit aspects of the information provided, or accepting that the knowledge used during the course of action may diverge from that presented in the documents, or that such knowledge evolves in situ (improvisation), based on an overarching objective provided by the prescribers.

Naturally, more than being two distinct types of content design, exhaustiveness and selectivity constitute two poles of the same dimension, which is the quantity of information provided directly by the cognitive aid. To make this design choice, *the cognitive aid must be perceived as a genuine information system capable of processing the requisite information (exhaustiveness) and adequate information (selectivity) to support the execution of a task in a relevant manner.* In this second part, we will explore how the model of the Turing machine offers a solution to approach a cognitive aid in this manner.

Cognitive aids as Turing machines

How can we explain that every cognitive aid is an information system, ranging from something as simple as a paper list to something as sophisticated as AI? Designing a cognitive aid involves creating an information system, and in this regard, the Turing machine emerges as a fitting model to capture this essential aspect. A Turing machine serves as both a universal and abstract information processing mechanism, while also providing a description of a contingent information processing scenario, which ultimately exhibits remarkable concreteness and simplicity. The Turing machine enables the description of diverse phenomena, from a knot in a handkerchief to the deductions of an inference engine, encompassing both the overarching principles of a cognitive aid and its operation within a specific context.

In a 1936 article, the British mathematician Alan Turing, one of the founding figures of what would later become computer science, delved into the essential, necessary and sufficient principles for describing an information processing system (Turing 1936). What particularly interests us here is the originality of his propositions, which describe very general and abstract principles through the lens of... cognitive aid usage. In simple terms, the Turing machine comprises an agent (either an individual or a machine) equipped with a tape, a pencil and an eraser. The tape is divided into a sequence of squares, each capable of holding a symbol from a predefined lexicon. On this tape, the agent can perform basic operations of writing and reading symbols. These operations include the following:

– Read the symbol displayed on a square of the tape.

– Write a symbol in a square. If a symbol is already present in this square, it will be erased and replaced by the new symbol.

– Move the tape from one square to another. The agent is equipped with a "reading head" (its field of perception and action) that points to a specific square at any given time.

– Between performing these operations, the agent is in a "mental state". As soon as the agent performs reading, writing or moving operations on the tape, the agent's mental state may change or remain in the same state. The significance of these mental states lies in their ability to interpret the same symbol on the tape in different ways. Depending on the agent's current state, reading the same symbol will have a specific meaning, leading to particular reading, writing or moving operations on the tape. Therefore, the symbol *S1* read in state *e1* will not have the same consequences as if the same symbol is read in state *e2*.

From this scenario that delineates the components of a Turing machine, it becomes feasible to program the execution of a task to be performed by the agent. Figure I2.2 illustrates the program for a rudimentary task outlined as follows: "If (mental state *e1* + reading of symbol *S1* on the tape) then (write symbol *S2* in place of *S1* + move to the right square + transition to state *e2*)". This directive will only be activated when the agent is in state *e1* and its reading head is positioned on a square containing the symbol *S1*, as depicted in Figure I2.2. Subsequently, upon examining the tape, we can predict that once this instruction is executed, the agent will be poised to read symbol *S3*, given that its reading head will be aligned with the square immediately to the right of the one containing symbol *S1*. In light of this new configuration, a fresh instruction could be drafted to guide the agent through the operations involving symbol *S3* in mental state *e2*.

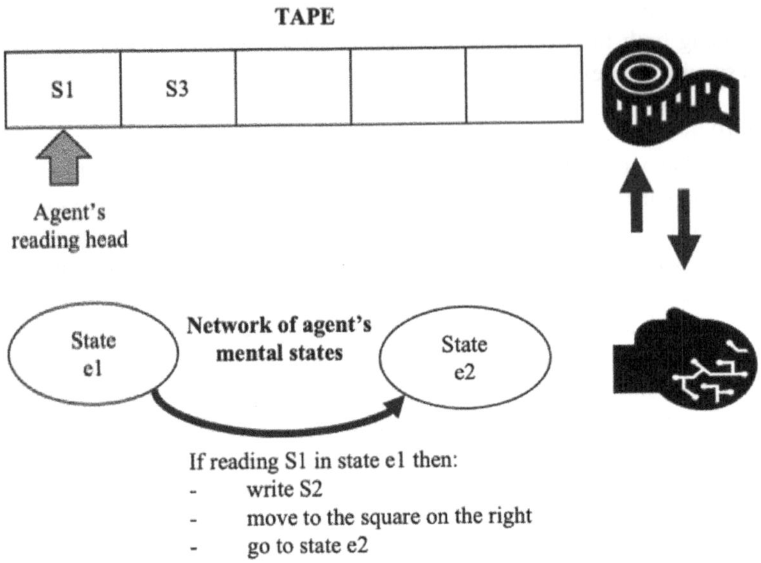

Figure I2.2. *Example of instructions for a Turing machine that writes symbol S2 in place of symbol S1 and continues its progression towards the square on the right, passing through states e1 and then e2*

Interestingly, the use of a cognitive aid can be described through this formalism. Returning to the previous example and considering that the tape in question is a handkerchief, this abstract program could be interpreted as describing the use of a knot in one's handkerchief as a mnemonic device. The program instructions could then be interpreted as follows:

– look at one's handkerchief (mental state *e1*);

– perceive a knot (symbol *S1* read);

– untie the knot (write symbol *S2* in place of *S1*);

– check if another knot is present (move to the square on the right);

– acknowledge the presence of this knot through recollection (state *e2*).

While computing was built on the basis of Turing's machines to conceptualize the internal architecture of a computer (where the tape represents the internal memory of the machine), it is noteworthy that, fundamentally, the information processing scenario described by Turing corresponds to an interaction between, on the one side, an agent and its mental operations, and on the other side, the external environment through the tape. In other words, it describes the functioning of a cognitive system. This aspect has been emphasized by some authors such as Wells (2004). Returning to this factual depiction of the situation envisioned by Turing, the Turing machine is essentially the manipulation by an agent of a "to-do list"! More precisely (and seriously), this formalism allows for the consideration of two types of *cognitive aids:*

– *cognitive aids that resemble a tape* (like a list, a checklist, for example);

– *cognitive aids that resemble a series of instructions for a network of mental states* (like a flowchart, a communication protocol dictating a sequence of information to be transmitted, for example).

Once the model of the Turing machine has been established to understand a cognitive aid, we can consider:

– the information content of the tape serving as a cognitive aid;

– the material form of the tape (the documentary medium);

– the network of mental states and the mental states involved;

– the transitions between these states with associated operations.

An analysis of the work should be able to provide answers to these questions.

TMTA: a work analysis method based on Turing machines

To devise a cognitive aid, the Turing machine model serves as a heuristic framework for the initial phase of needs assessment through work analysis. This is demonstrated by the Turing Machine Task Analysis (TMTA) method (Morineau et al. 2009b; Morineau 2010, 2011). This method comprises two main stages.

– *Work domain analysis: this involves analyzing the environment in which operators operate, an environment that presents them with constraints and action possibilities.*

– *Task analysis: this involves analyzing the goals and operations assigned to the agent for execution, which can be depicted as a network of states.*

The *work domain* broadly encompasses *the objects on which operators perform tasks*. In the field of healthcare, the central object is undoubtedly the patient, approached from the perspective of biomedical knowledge, anatomy and physiology. However, other objects also exist in this domain, such as technological devices, equipment, medical instruments and supplies used by healthcare providers. These objects impose peripheral tasks on operators.

Task analysis involves describing, in a formal manner, *the objectives to be achieved by operators and the sub-steps they must take to reach these objectives.* Ultimately, the interaction between the objects within the work domain and a sequence of goals and subgoals to be achieved corresponds to a work situation. These two steps of the TMTA method draw inspiration from cognitive engineering studies, leading to a reflection on work organization, strategies employed by operators, and the skills they must use. Together, these analytical stages form what is known as *cognitive work analysis* (Vicente 1999).

In the two chapters of this second part, we will respectively present the following:

– work domain analysis, which proves to be a suitable methodological framework for designing cognitive aids that integrate into the work environment, thus easily likened to Turing machine tapes;

– task analysis, which is more suitable for designing cognitive aids guiding cognitive operations, thus resembling networks of Turing machine states.

However, it should be noted that beyond this somewhat arbitrary separation necessary for exposition, these two types of analysis (domain and task) can complement each other in designing a particular cognitive aid. Moreover, any cognitive aid can ultimately be understood from one of these two perspectives (tape or state network).

6

Analyzing the Work Domain to Design a Tape

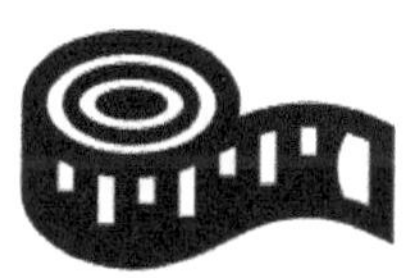

Figure 6.1. *The tape of a Turing machine*

Many cognitive aids can be easily likened to the tape of a Turing machine. Whether it is a set of items written, crossed out, or annotated on a sheet of paper or a whiteboard, columns in a table detailing categorized data, or even a page in an agenda, these are all cognitive aids that can be conceptualized in a similar manner. They possess a physical medium, compartments and symbols within those compartments. In the field of aeronautics, the resemblance between cognitive aids and Turing machine tape can be particularly striking. For instance, the scroll checklist used in older military aircraft models is essentially a tape inserted into a physical mechanism that enables vertical scrolling when the user manipulates the two knobs on the sides of the device. This scrolling mechanism facilitates transitioning from one item to another (see Figure 6.2).

In the medical field, a prime example of a cognitive aid that truly resembles a tape marked with compartments is the Broselow tape. This tape is used by SMUR teams during out-of-hospital interventions with children. Unfurled along the length of the supine child, the tape features centimeter measurements paired with crucial information for management, including estimated weight, typical medication dosages and expected values for certain physiological parameters such as heart rate and respiratory rate, all tailored to the child's height.

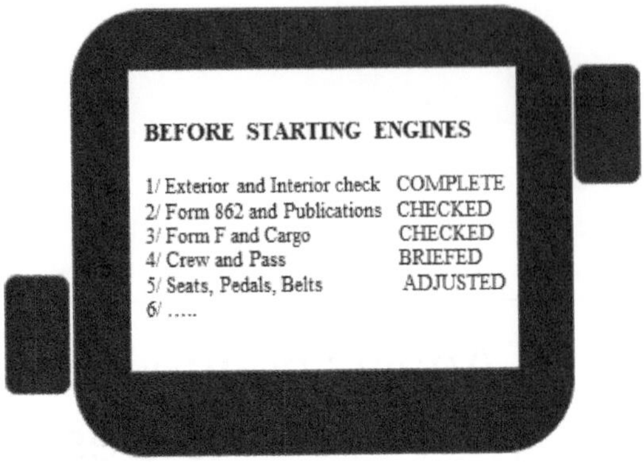

Figure 6.2. *An old "scroll-out" checklist with two joysticks, aboard US military aircraft*[1]

In a design context, a central question is to define the information content, as well as the material form of the tape, ergonomically, i.e. according to the constraints of the work situation. The analysis of the work domain describes the objects on which the work focuses. *The premise of the work domain analysis is that it is necessary for the cognitive aid to reflect the objects and properties of the domain in order to provide support to operators*. The cognitive aid should be able to highlight certain important aspects of the work environment that need to be considered when performing tasks in this environment. Using our terminology, this amounts to designing a gateway between the work environment and the operators' cognition. This is the logic underlying what is referred to in cognitive engineering systems as ecological interface design (Vicente and Rasmussen 1992; Burns and Hajdukiewicz 2017). An illustration will concretize this logic of reflecting the work domain through a human–machine interface, via a cognitive aid.

6.1. An ecological interface for supervising an emergency service department

The concept of ecological interface has been used to redesign the information content of patient flow supervision software within an emergency department (McGeorge et al. 2015). Here, the domain is not the patient directly, but rather a group of patients managed by a team of caregivers within a department. By conducting a work domain analysis, the researchers aimed to:

– represent patients according to the phases of their management;

1 See: https://www.usmilitariaforum.com.

– assist in rapidly assessing the number of patients awaiting care, based on their severity level;

– aid in identifying bottlenecks in the flow (unusual waiting times for examinations, delays in patient reassessment);

– help balance the workload among caregivers.

Two software applications were evaluated. The first resembled the one typically used in the service. It presented the information in a tabular format with columnar variables, such as the treatment room, patient's name, age/gender, reason for visit, arrival time, attending physicians and nurses, vital signs, additional examinations and comments. The list of patients present in the ward constituted the rows of this table, composed of alphanumeric sequences. In essence, it resembled a conventional Excel spreadsheet, visually similar to a basic tape. The second software interface was a prototype design based on the analysis of the work domain. Eight key variables were represented through graphs, presenting the information in both a synthetic and schematic manner.

– Patients in the waiting room: a histogram showing their number, severity level and waiting time.

– Patient flow: curves describing the evolution of the number of patients according to the stage in their management (five predefined stages).

– A star graph presenting a general overview of key indicators: number of patients in different stages of care, average time for the first assessment by a doctor and average time of patient presence in the service.

– A graph composed of colored dots indicating bed status (available, unavailable or occupied) and, if occupied, the duration and care stage of the patient.

– A histogram showing queues and waiting times for additional examinations.

– A histogram providing an estimate of caregivers' workload based on the number of patients each cares for and the severity of their condition.

– A table presented in a classical manner, with added graph bars indicating the time spent by each patient in each stage of their care.

All of these psychological instruments were presented on a single screen, allowing for a comprehensive view of the situation, in line with the principles guiding the design of ecological interfaces.

An evaluation of these two interfaces in a simulation center equipped with a series of patient-simulation mannequins and conducted among 14 pairs of "physician–nurse" emergency caregivers showed, through subjective assessment, that the new display based on the principle of ecological interfaces provided better support for cognitive activity, without imposing a significant additional mental burden. However, this new software was unfamiliar to the participants and had not benefited from a period of familiarization.

Beyond the ease of perception provided by the graphs constituting an ecological interface, the representation of high-level variables of significance (chunks) reflecting the most abstract levels of a work domain prevents the operators from exerting mental effort to understand the situation. For example, the abstract notion of caregiver workload in the ward is presented in the ecological interface in a directly accessible way. Accessing this notion with the old software would have required significant mental calculation, repeated with every glance at the interface.

6.2. The techniques of work domain analysis

Domain analysis as the first step in work analysis is a peculiarity stemming from the field of cognitive systems engineering, pioneered by Danish researcher Rasmussen (1985), whose work led to the development of Cognitive Work Analysis by Vicente (1999). The TMTA method incorporates this initial domain analysis step by integrating the framework of Turing machines.

While traditional methods of work analysis, especially those in French-speaking contexts, often begin with an analysis of operators' task sequences, cognitive engineering emphasizes the importance of *starting with an ontological description of the work environment's reality. This reality fundamentally explains the presence of operators, who have tasks necessary for domain control.* Therefore, the work of nurses, doctors or nursing assistants cannot be understood without fundamental reference to the notion of patient care, which plays a decisive role in defining the constraints caregivers face in their tasks. For example, patients requiring palliative care impose a significant psychological burden due to frequent encounters with death. Another context is road accidents, which require SMUR teams to adapt to highly variable and sometimes very challenging physical environments. Designing an adapted cognitive aid involves consideration of these specific constraints of a work domain. *If we initially consider the goals to be achieved through task analysis, we may find caregivers with similar goals but operating in vastly different work environments, with constraints rendering the situations incomparable.* It is worth noting that modeling hospital management processes carries the same risk of contextualizing effective activity; ultimately, processes roughly correspond to tasks.

While the constraints of a work domain can be described in different ways, the original technique proposed by Rasmussen is the *abstraction hierarchy*. However, before delving into this technique, it is essential to emphasize the importance, in this initial step of work analysis, of delineating the domain.

6.2.1. *Delineating the work domain*

The description of the environment within which agents carry out operations can vary greatly depending on one's perspective of this environment. Indeed, a work domain is a subset of the overall environment and the precise delineation of this part of the environment always remains arbitrary. For instance, providing care for a patient may involve more than just improving their physiological condition; it may also impact their psychological well-being, their family, loved ones and the organizations they are part of, such as their workplace or even the healthcare system itself. During a work analysis, it is crucial to delimit the relevant domain to avoid making the subject of study too broad or ambiguous to be meaningfully addressed. In the context of designing a cognitive aid, this delimitation will be determined by its intended purposes. The delimitation of the domain will need to be considered in terms of breadth, depth, time and the operators involved.

– *Breadth delimitation.* Where does the domain to be considered for designing a cognitive aid end or, in other words, which elements of the environment will be affected by its functions? In the study by Dryver et al. (2021) described in Chapter 1, it is demonstrated that the developed cognitive aid significantly improved adherence to the steps in managing a clinical case. However, this aid did not address the preliminary diagnostic phase; it lacked this functionality. Ideally, it would have been interesting (and more ambitious) to broaden the scope by including the medical diagnosis stage. Similarly, should cognitive support for the management of polytrauma patients be restricted to personnel and tasks within the vital emergency reception area or should it encompass communications with the out-of-hospital team that attended to the victim? The broader the domain covered by the assistance, the greater its integrative value and thus its utility (exhaustiveness); however, the risk is increased complexity and decreased ease of use, necessitating selectivity.

– *Depth delimitation.* Once the boundaries of the domain are defined, it is necessary to consider the level of granularity within the domain that will be described. For example, should a resuscitation aid focus solely on recalling the different stages of the procedure to be followed or should it also provide assistance in carrying out specific technical procedures, such as assisting with the intubation procedure or calculating and preparing doses? Similar to domain breadth delimitation, a compromise between exhaustiveness and selectivity will be necessary.

– *Temporal delimitation.* The domain is not only a spatial concept but also a temporal interval during which cognitive aid must be able to support teams. For instance, when considering patient care in terms of a "patient journey" and facilitating coordination among various medical and medico-social actors, the time interval can be extensive but remains relevant at the patient level. In particular, with the growing prominence of outpatient care and telemedicine, there is a need to extend the scope of patient care beyond the duration of their stay in a department.

– *Delimitation of the operators involved.* Finally, the description of a work domain is based on the perspectives of a group of operators who need to intervene in this domain. A patient will be viewed from a specific angle, depending on whether they are undergoing diagnosis, treatment or personal care. Therefore, it is crucial to specify the categories of operators for whom the description of the domain will be relevant.

6.2.2. *Abstraction hierarchy*

The abstraction hierarchy is the primary technique of explication, proposed by cognitive engineering, for describing all the objects comprising a work domain. *Through an abstraction hierarchy, the objects of the domain, as concrete physical forms, are also described in terms of functions, processes they contribute to, abstract functions (core principles and fundamental laws of the domain), and functional goals enabled by these objects*. This results in a table in which the rows represent various viewpoints, ranging from more concrete to more abstract, on the objects within the work domain (Box 6.1).

The five levels of an abstraction hierarchy, ranging from the most abstract to the most concrete, illustrated using the human body as a work domain.

– *Functional goals* represent the essential objectives associated with controlling the work domain (such as the organism's adaptive responses).

– *Abstract functions* represent the general principles governing the work domain or the fundamental criteria for considering the domain (such as the laws governing normal and pathological cellular functioning).

– *Processes* (also referred to as *generalized functions*) involve physical forms and their functions (such as the physiological systems of the body like the endocrine system, the cardiovascular system, etc.).

– *Physical functions* performed by these physical forms (such as the physiological functioning of organs).

– *Physical forms and tangible appearances* of objects perceivable in the domain (such as the anatomy of the patient).

Box 6.1. *The different levels of an abstraction hierarchy*

The table presenting an abstraction hierarchy typically consists of five rows, representing five perspectives on the domain, which constitute an abstraction hierarchy. Functional relationships of the "means-to-ends" type between the different perspectives can be elucidated. Through these relationships, the lower (concrete) levels of the hierarchy of abstraction serve as means to achieve the higher (abstract) levels, which are the ends to be attained.

When the domain is complex, it is possible to decompose it into subunits and create an abstraction hierarchy for each of these components. In this case, the table is divided into columns (Figure 6.3). These columns represent a *"part-whole" or aggregation hierarchy*. Each column represents a structural level of the domain, with its own abstraction hierarchy in rows.

Table 6.1 is a simplified example of an abstraction hierarchy used to describe the domain of diagnosing abdominal pain. The purpose of this work was to initiate a process to identify the assistance needs that astronauts might have in a space base during a medical emergency. As these astronauts are not necessarily doctors, the scope of assistance involves tele-expertise provided by a medical doctor on Earth, which can be supplemented by onsite assistance software (Bernard et al. 2021). Given the distance of the communication, the objective was to establish a framework to define the necessary yet sufficient information needs in healthcare contexts. Based on this scenario and a collection of medical information, an initial abstraction hierarchy was developed.

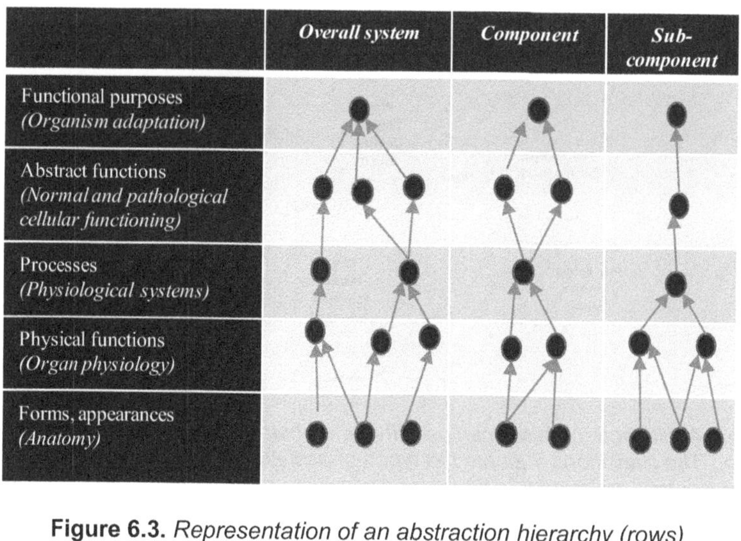

Figure 6.3. *Representation of an abstraction hierarchy (rows) and an aggregation hierarchy (columns). The example of the human body is presented in parentheses and italics*

Functional purposes	Diagnosis of abdominal pain		
Abstract functions	Non-serious appendicitis; generalized peritonitis; simple prostatitis; simple gastroenteritis; peritonitis; carbon monoxide poisoning, etc.		
Processes	Physiological parameters: heart rate, blood pressure, oxygen saturation	Medical history: location, intensity, time of last meal, nausea, vomiting, diarrhea, urinary signs, headaches, onset of symptoms	Quadrants (abdominal areas), pain, rigidity
Physical functions	Monitoring a patient	Responses, questions	Palpation
Physical forms	Equipment: physiological monitor, sensors, user interfaces	Equipment: oral or written questionnaire	Position and location of hands

Table 6.1. *Abstraction hierarchy describing the diagnosis of abdominal pain. The "means-to-ends" links are not described (Bernard et al. 2021)*

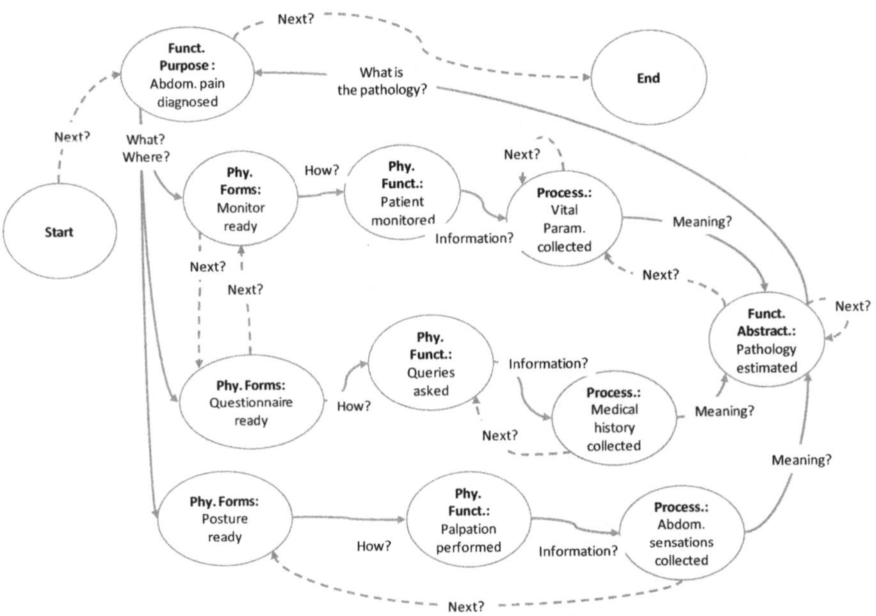

Figure 6.4. *Network of relationships within the abstraction hierarchy for "abdominal pain". The transitions indicate the types of assistance that may be necessary. For a color version of this figure, see www.iste.co.uk/morineau/cognitive.zip*

Figure 6.4 presents the "means–end" relationships that may exist between the levels of the abstraction hierarchy in Table 6.1, concerning the domain of abdominal pain. Three paths are identifiable in this network: the first concerns the monitoring of the patient's physiological parameters, the second involves using a questionnaire administered to the patient regarding their symptoms and recent meals, and the third path involves abdominal palpation to locate and characterize pain. These relationships highlight the types of information that novice caregivers are likely to request, either from the remote expert or from the available cognitive assistance on site (paper document or software). It is worth noting that representing this type of network can quickly lead to modeling in terms of a state network for a Turing machine.

More specifically, this "means-to-ends" network related to abdominal pain highlights various types of information that may be required in assistance, depending on the levels of abstraction in the hierarchy:

– the location of equipment (monitor, questionnaire);

– the operating procedure for using the physiological monitor, the questionnaire or performing palpations;

– the relevant information to consider;

– their interpretation to access their meaning;

– assistance in decision-making by providing a diagnostic result.

To design an abstraction hierarchy, various sources of information (domain documents, interviews with experts) can be used. Alternatively, the following technique for defining the content of cognitive aid focuses on expert consultation.

6.2.3. *The Delphi technique: consulting domain experts*

The Delphi technique facilitates consultation of experts on a specific topic. Accordingly, it can be used to define the items of a cognitive aid. Several steps are involved (ORSAS Lorraine 2009).

– Step 1: define the object of inquiry precisely and rigorously. Similar to what was previously indicated, this involves accurately describing the field to which the desired assistance pertains, the objectives of the device and the conditions of its use. The broad dimensions used to understand the exhaustiveness and selectivity of the content, as discussed earlier, can contribute to this initial step (distribution of internal/external cognition balance between intuition and analysis, degree of alignment between task and actual activity).

– Step 2: selection of experts. They must possess expertise in the relevant field while also being representative and independent.

– Step 3: development of a questionnaire for the experts. It is crucial to present precise and targeted questions to the panel, adhering to recommendations on questionnaire construction to mitigate response biases (such as question-affirmative sentences that may generate a positive response). This questionnaire will be individually distributed to each expert.

– Step 4: administration of the questionnaire in four rounds. Following an initial individual round, the results of the questions and comments from the first round are shared with the experts for reconsideration, taking into account the overall responses from the panel. If some experts propose new answers that differ significantly from the majority, they must provide justification (using median and quartiles for quantifying results). This iterative process continues until the 4th and final round, during which all data from preceding rounds are presented to the panel for a conclusive evaluation, leading to definitive responses. The data will then be processed and synthesized into a final report.

An example of using the Delphi method to develop a cognitive aid is the creation of a checklist for verifying electronic drug prescriptions for interns and young practitioners (Desnoyer et al. 2017). The aim of this aid was to prevent the creation of incorrect prescriptions. The overall design process comprised five steps:

– selection of medical experts;

– literature review;

– conducting 17 semi-structured interviews with experts;

– conducting two rounds of Delphi;

– translation of items into English;

– development of the software tool.

During this design process, 40 doctors and 25 pharmacists participated in the study, representing 22 universities and hospitals across four countries: Canada, Belgium, France and Switzerland. While 166 items emerged after the literature review, the final checklist, following the application of the Delphi method, comprised 160 items integrated into the software.

The abstraction hierarchy and the Delphi method enable exhaustive exploration of the information content of a cognitive aid. However, once the domain has been thoroughly examined, specific constraints related to the contexts in which aid is used must be posed to achieve greater selectivity.

6.2.4. *Constraints on the content of a cognitive aid*

In line with the issue of the relevance of cognitive aids, Degani and Wiener (1990), in their study report commissioned by NASA on aviation checklists, underscore the tension between exhaustiveness and selectivity. Managing these two demands is crucial to ensure that the tape displays the necessary squares and symbols (exhaustiveness) while being sufficient (selectivity) to guide the course of the activity. The primary design challenge is therefore to define what constitutes relevant information in a specific context. Following the guidelines of the aviation domain, the American ATA (Air Transport Association) has proposed the following principle for designing flight checklists.

> Checklists should contain, in abbreviated form, all the information required by the trained flight crew to operate the airplane in most normal and non-normal situations. Normal check-lists should be organized by segments of flight. The checklist should contain the minimum cues required for the trained crew-member to verify that the appropriate actions have been completed. Only procedural steps which, if omitted have direct and adverse impact on normal operations, are included. Items annunciated by crew alerting systems are not included (Degani and Wiener 1990).

In aviation, critical items are referred to as *killer items*. To define these critical items, which we would characterize as *relevant items* in the strict sense proposed by the theory of relevance, it is possible to use the model of the Turing machine.

Let us consider the example of a checklist. It will be represented by a tape. Each square on this tape corresponds to an item on the checklist. Every symbol read or written in each square represents the verification of the checklist by the operator (the agent). To identify the necessary and sufficient items, it will be necessary to define the squares and symbols that enable the agent to progress through their network of mental states until they accomplish the overall verification task. In other words, if we have the sequence of states that the agent must pass through (the task to be completed), we can deduce the squares and symbols on the tape that facilitate transitions from one state to another in this network. Therefore, we should obtain the necessary and sufficient information to be represented in the checklist.

Let us consider the design of a checklist for the management of a life-threatening emergency following the ABCDE protocol (Peran et al. 2020). It is important to note that the letters ABCDE signify the need to diagnose and manage the patient by following the sequence of steps: Airway (ensure the airway is clear), Breathing (ensure adequate breathing), Circulation (assess circulatory status), Disability (evaluate level of consciousness) and Exposure (check for hemorrhage and trauma).

The caregiver must identify the necessary and sufficient indicators to ensure that each step is achieved, thereby confirming the transition to the next stage of the procedure. For instance, the agent marks the symbol "OK" on the square labeled "Position of the head facilitating breathing" in the Airway state when perceiving indicators in the situation that validate this state, enabling progression to the next stage, Breathing.

As shown in Figure 6.4, illustrating a Turing model for this procedure, the task at hand is to select the critical indicators (squares on the tape) observable from the patient, which must trigger the transition to the next step. The state network of the Turing machine is interpreted as follows:

– "In state A (airway), if there are indications confirming airway clearance, then mark the square (OK), move to the adjacent square, and transition to state B".

– "If no indications are present (No), then take action to clear the airway and remain in state A". This action cycles back to state A, indicating that the process of clearing the airway must be repeated until the symbol "OK" is marked on the tape.

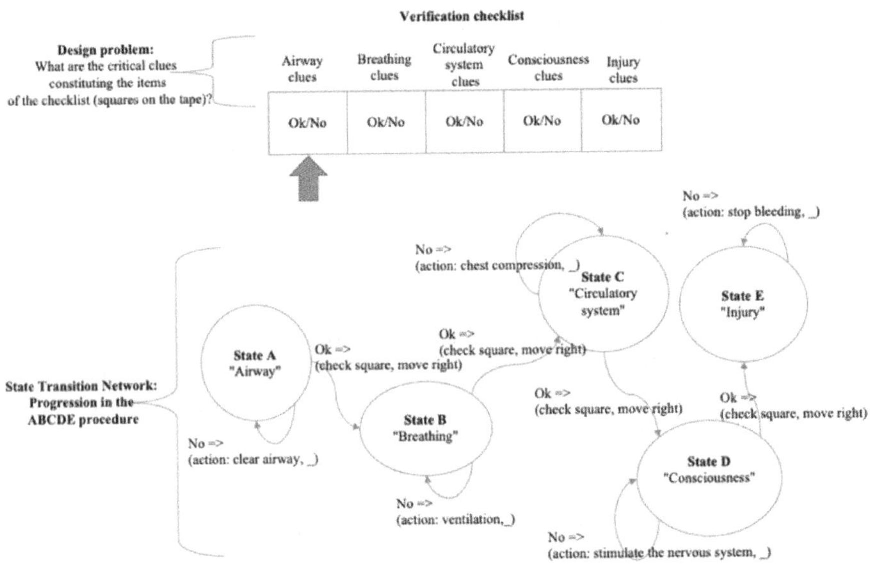

Figure 6.5. *Turing machine modeling of the search for clues to conduct an ABCDE protocol for the care of a patient in an emergency situation*

Figure 6.5 does not provide the necessary and sufficient clues to allow the transition between the ABCDE mental states: this is the solution to the checklist design problem. This model “only” formalizes the problem, thus allowing for the structuring of the search for clues to be presented on the checklist in a rigorous manner. Once these clues (squares) are identified, it will be possible to simulate the operation of the Turing machine and thus ensure that the agent can effectively progress to state E. This formalization effort also shows the limitations of a protocol. Here, its highly sequential nature means that the presence of a hemorrhagic wound is only addressed last, which may not be suitable in actual activity. Sequencing a series of care through a protocol like ABCDE means choosing a prioritization of actions to be taken, which corresponds to a form of selection. In reality, patient care may prioritize the treatment of a hemorrhage or involve a team capable of treating various resuscitation steps in parallel. The protocol will not be strictly followed. Turing machine modeling accurately describes the task as envisioned by the prescribers. *In a protocol evaluation process, this formalization can serve as a reference for understanding the deviations observed in actual activity*. This may potentially lead to the evolution of cognitive aids to better align with the real constraints of situations experienced by caregivers.

6.2.5. *Constraints on the material form of a cognitive aid*

Defined as a tape, a cognitive aid is primarily an object situated within a material environment and integrated into the perceptual-motor loops of its users. Much of the ease of use of the cognitive aid hinges on its physical attributes: shape, volume, weight, necessary accessories, energy and consumable requirements (such as paper and ink for writing or printing), size of the information display area allowing for varying degrees of sharing within a workgroup and level of technical complexity involving potentially vulnerable technology or technology requiring updates. These properties manifest as more or less facilitating *affordances* in different contexts of object manipulation.

Drawing on the ergonomics research of Richard (1990) and Sebillotte (1995), we have proposed to decompose the tasks of handling equipment and instruments – and thus the manipulation of cognitive aids – into three categories: prerequisites, corequisites and post-requisites (Morineau et al. 2016).

– *A prerequisite*: this involves a preliminary action to be completed before using a specific piece of equipment or entering a designated space. For instance, retrieving a medical instrument from a storage area. Depending on the environmental context, this preliminary action may vary in duration and complexity. If the instrument is within arm’s reach, simply grabbing it suffices. However, if it is stored in a medical cart, we must navigate to the cart, locate the correct drawer, open it and retrieve the item.

– *A corequisite*: this involves actions necessary for controlling the object during its use, such as ensuring a urinary catheter does not leak while being inserted. These corequisites are peripheral actions subject to attentional control and supervision, yet they are crucial to achieving the desired goal.

– *A post-requisite*: this pertains to an action to be performed after obtaining the result of the initial action. For example, returning an instrument to a designated location in a suitable condition for preservation and easy retrieval. Activities related to organization and storage fulfill the requirements of post-requisites.

Table 6.2 presents, for illustrative purposes, a comparison between three types of documentary media (paper notebook, digital tablet, large fixed screen) for cognitive aids, considering their points of fragility (in gray) regarding a set of prerequisites, corequisites and post-requisites.

In terms of prerequisites, a digital tablet is a fragile device that requires a dedicated storage area. A paper notebook can be easily moved during use like a digital tablet. However, the fixed screen remains stationary. Both the notebook and the tablet are easy to place on another support. Mounting a large screen requires a wall with a sufficiently sized surface or a telescopic arm, which can be cumbersome. In addition, digital devices such as the tablet and screen require electrical connection or rechargeable batteries. Conversely, the notebook consumes paper resources. Before their effective use, digital devices require actions such as powering on, password authentication and software updates, which can significantly prolong processing times, especially when the computer network lacks sufficient power. For example, during the observation of a crisis management simulation exercise, an observer noted a wait of up to 7 minutes before the various software programs on the crisis team's computers could be used.

In terms of corequisites, digital supports involve navigation systems within the software. The fixed large screen does not allow for mobility. However, the mobility afforded by the digital tablet also makes it fragile, which is not the case for paper support. As both the notebook and the tablet are mobile, they require stable support to be used easily. During use, all three supports are difficult to share in order for multiple users to write on the document. A whiteboard would be more suitable for such functionality. This is also true for shared reading, except for the large screen, whose information sharing capability is a major function. Finally, if the information content is dense, the notebook will require numerous pages with the potential need for a table of contents, which would slow down access to information. The document would also be physically larger. Conversely, digital terminals allow for rapid access to information through icons or a search bar if they have been designed ergonomically. Their physical volume is not dependent on the quantity of information contained.

	Paper notebook	Digital tablet	Large fixed screen
Prerequisites			
Retrieve from storage			
Move			
Place on another support			
Power			
Supply consumables			
Prepare for use (power on, login, updates)			
Corequisites			
Peripheral information to process			
Mobility during use			
Durability during use			
Maintain device position			
Share content in writing			
Share content in reading			
Scroll through content			
Post-requisites			
Store			
Protect			
Clean, disinfect			
Dispose			
Repair			

Table 6.2. *Comparative illustration of three documentary supports based on prerequisites, corequisites and post-requisites. Gray-colored cells represent the points of fragility of the three supports*

Once used, each type of support requires postliminary actions, known as post-requisites, to be fulfilled. Tablets can be misplaced and are fragile, requiring storage and protection. Digital technologies are more challenging to repair or dispose of compared to a paper notebook. These represent significant investments, and even in the event of malfunctions, such as delays in accessing data, immediate replacement may not occur. Conversely, cleaning is a weak point in paper usage.

This framework for delineating actions surrounding the use of a documentary device can be employed to evaluate different solutions proposed for the development of cognitive aids. Besides clarifying these constraints, trials with potential users in real or simulated work settings will uncover hidden affordances, such as a control button that is difficult to perceive on a support, or false affordances, where users believe a function is activated through touch when it requires pressing a button. Streamlining all peripheral actions related to a documentary medium helps to reduce the number of constraints faced by operators. If a cognitive aid imposes more constraints than supportive functions, it risks being quickly abandoned.

Despite criticism for being a method that seeks to maximize productivity, the LEAN method is compelling as it aims to reduce the number of prerequisites, corequisites and post-requisites, allowing operators to focus solely on core business actions. This approach frees up time for practitioners, potentially improving patient management. The LEAN method targets optimization of the preparation, maintenance and storage of equipment and supplies. Originating from the industrial sector, particularly the automotive domain with the Toyota Production System model, the method was revisited by MIT in the 1980s. Following extensive adoption in the industrial realm, initial applications in the hospital setting emerged in the 2000s in anglophone countries, later spreading to France. The LEAN method involves conducting an inventory of equipment and supplies and mapping movement flows to access these resources, typically performed collaboratively with users.

The 5S technique comprises the following:

– *Sorting* products by eliminating those whose expiration date has passed.

– *Setting up* storage areas by improving organization for easy understanding and use (e.g. placing heavy products on lower shelves for accessibility and adopting visual management principles where relevant products are visible within 3 seconds).

– *Shining* surfaces to disinfect them, enhance the usability of work areas and reduce the informational clutter caused by the presence of waste.

– *Standardizing* storage methods to facilitate understanding and implementing this new procedure throughout the department.

– *Sustaining* regular checks over time to monitor the evolution of operating methods and adapt them as needed.

Box 6.2. *The 5S technique in the LEAN method*

After conducting this diagnosis, the next step is to reorganize the storage areas using the *5S technique* (Venkateswaran et al. 2013). This 5S technique can be applied to cognitive aids to optimize prerequisites, corequisites and post-requisites. However, it can also lead to regarding the work environment, in its entirety, as a cognitive aid in itself. Therefore, *the work environment per se can be seen as a collection of cognitive aids, particularly if it is conceived as a space in which cognition is distributed.* The work environment then becomes a generalized Turing machine tape.

6.2.6. *Part of the environment as a cognitive aid: a triage station in the emergency department*

In a work environment, a simple table used for placing files on can become a significant cognitive aid if it is reimagined as a space where a portion of cognition is redistributed (distributed cognition). At the emergency reception of a hospital we collaborated with, the administrative registration of a patient is carried out by a medical administrative assistant. A digital file and a paper file (a Kraft envelope) are prepared for each patient. Subsequently, the paper file is placed on a table situated between the assistant and the triage nurse. The nurse then takes the file to supplement it with clinical data. The paper files are arranged on the table in order of arrival, implicitly corresponding to a prioritization criterion for patient management. The first patient to arrive should ideally be attended to first, except in cases of absolute urgency. Subsequently, their actual medical care by the medical teams will be based on severity level, measured during the triage activity by the nurse. Furthermore, considering that there are (at the time) two main care zones in the department – the “medical” zone for individuals with medical conditions and the “traumatology” zone for individuals with injuries or fractures – each file envelope is manually marked with a letter indicating the targeted zone (*M* for medical, *T* for traumatology, or another letter if the file concerns another zone, such as a gynecological consultation – to simplify the modeling of the problem, we will use the letter *A* for “Other zone”).

Figure 6.6 shows the table and its contents before the ergonomic intervention. It is noteworthy that, in addition to the patient files, tools and equipment are stored on the table. The table appears as a common affordance, encouraging the placement of any objects required to be within reach of healthcare providers for their activities (e.g. gloves, hand sanitizer, documents, etc.).

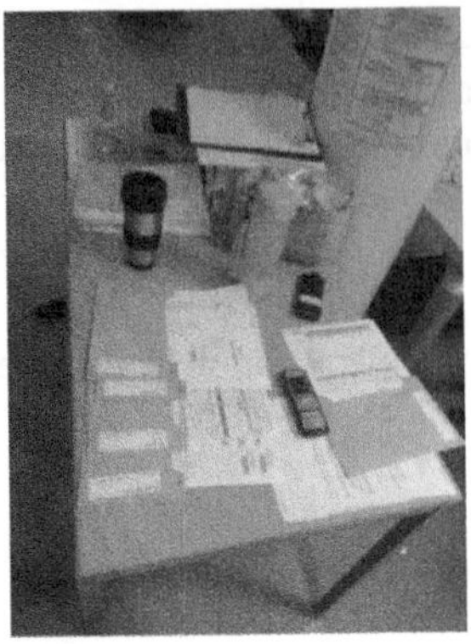

Figure 6.6. *Table for depositing "patient" files at the emergency reception, before the ergonomic intervention (reproduction authorized: Bretagne Atlantique Hospital Center). For a color version of this figure, see www.iste.co.uk/morineau/cognitive.zip*

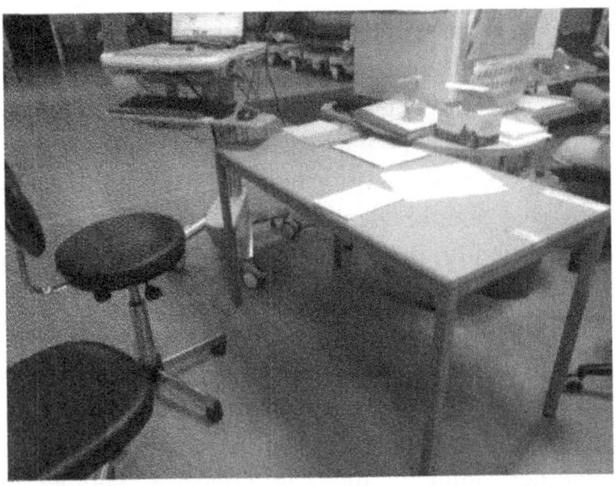

Figure 6.7. *Table for depositing "patient" files at the emergency reception, after ergonomic intervention (reproduction authorized: Bretagne Atlantique Hospital Center). For a color version of this figure, see www.iste.co.uk/morineau/cognitive.zip*

We understand that affordance-driven behaviors stem from intuitive thinking (system 1). Therefore, tracking the evolution of the contents of this table over time reveals that the variety of stored objects and the manner in which files are placed generate informational noise and false affordances for the patient registration task. Particularly when arrivals multiply in the department, files accumulate, and the next "patient" file needing consideration is sometimes buried among disorderly objects. In terms of cognitive aids, the table fails to fully guide the caregiver in their actions, while the triage nurse's mental load reached in certain frequent situations would warrant allocating part of this burden to the external environment. Conversely, the table contributes to the surrounding informational noise, exacerbating this workload.

Figure 6.7 shows how this table and its environment have been redesigned to constitute a tape belonging to an information system. Initially, the equipment was removed and placed on a shelf arranged next to the table to first eliminate informational noise. Subsequently, the table's space was divided into areas, or squares, resembling a Turing machine's tape. Initially, two squares were created, separated by a yellow line and each labeled to indicate the patient's zone (Medicine/Traumatology or Other zone). Later, based on an idea from a caregiver in the service (*participatory design*), a third small area was designated for specific cases.

This new configuration facilitates file categorization. Without needing to search for the letter on the envelope, the nurse can directly identify the area to refer the patient to. Figures 6.8 and 6.9 depict file processing on the table, respectively showing a single queue (previous situation) or two queues (newly created situation). With two queues, *the Turing machine becomes non-deterministic, meaning its operation depends on the agent's decision*. The triage nurse thus has more degrees of freedom than when they are simply processing the next available file.

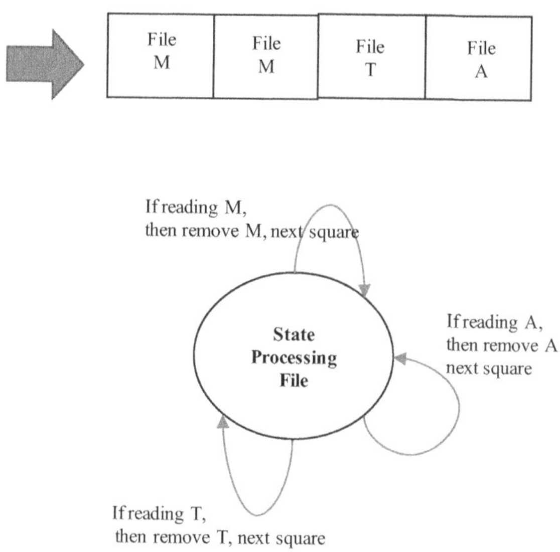

Figure 6.8. *Turing machine modeling file processing with a file queue, before ergonomic intervention*

With the presence of a single undifferentiated line, patients destined for different zones were previously mixed. However, due to the fact that there are very frequently a greater number of "medicine" files than "traumatology" files, this single queue led patients destined for traumatology to wait in the general queue, when they were perhaps the first to go to the traumatology department. From the point of view of the patient flow, this single queue thus created unnecessary expectations. With two queues, the first folder for medicine and that for traumatology are easily identifiable, and the nurse can choose to alternate the processing of files in each queue, in order to balance the flows to each zone. In addition to not making some patients wait unnecessarily, these two queues make it possible to evenly distribute the workload in the two sectors, through balanced arrival frequencies. This table, transformed into a component of a Turing machine, is no longer a simple table: it has become a work aid.

If this redesign has not been clearly explained through a technique such as abstraction hierarchy, the result still corresponds well to the desire for a better representation of the work domain in the equipment used by operators (the table). Indeed, peripheral objects (mask box, glove box, etc.) have been removed, and the essential constraints of the domain regarding the presence of the different zones to which patients are to be directed have been highlighted through the new layout of the table. In a way, the table has become an ecological interface, albeit frugal, but responding to the logic of directly reflecting the constraints of the domain through the assistance device.

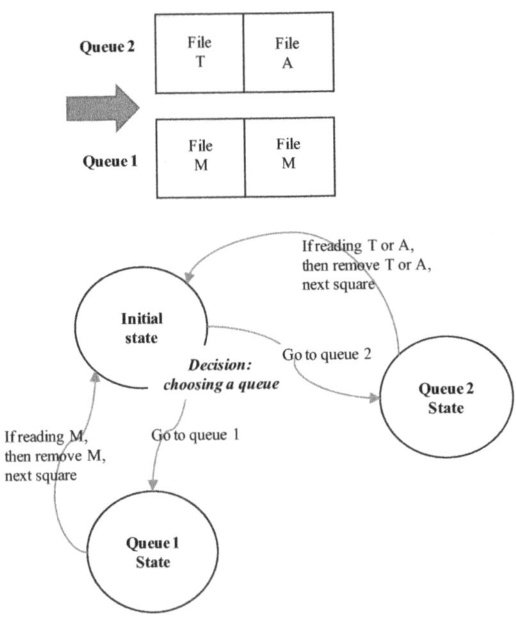

Figure 6.9. *Turing machine modeling the processing of files with two file queues after ergonomic intervention*

6.2.7. *Ergonomic evaluation tools for content and format*

The previous example of redesigning the layout of a table demonstrates the uniqueness of each workstation. In each case, the analyst must thoroughly understand the situation to consider its constraints and degrees of freedom before proposing ergonomic solutions.

Ergonomics has few general rules; it is primarily an empirical discipline. Nevertheless, there are some general recommendations for drafting working documents that serve as cognitive aids.

The Cognitive aids in Medicine Assessment Tool (CMAT) (Evans et al. 2015) provides a list of criteria for this purpose. It consists of a questionnaire with 42 items designed to evaluate the ergonomic qualities of a cognitive aid (see Figure 6.10). The recommendations are categorized into three main themes.

– *Physical characteristics of the document*: this includes aspects such as size, presence of tabs, font type and margins. Notably, this category directly involves an assessment of the affordances provided by the document medium.

– *Content structure*: this involves elements such as minimum content requirements, titles, identified potential deficiencies and points of vigilance.

– *Format and display*: this encompasses considerations such as page layout, beginning/end markers, incorporation of figures and tables, and use of abbreviations.

In addition, we can draw upon the recommendations provided by Brangier and Barcenilla (2001). These recommendations pertain to the drafting of working documents such as “manuals” or “user guides”. Their criteria are categorized into six themes:

– general presentation of the document and its structure;

– vocabulary usage and operative language (field-specific jargon to be employed);

– sentence construction;

– information content;

– safety instructions and specific guidance;

– recommendations regarding the use of illustrations (tables, diagrams, etc.).

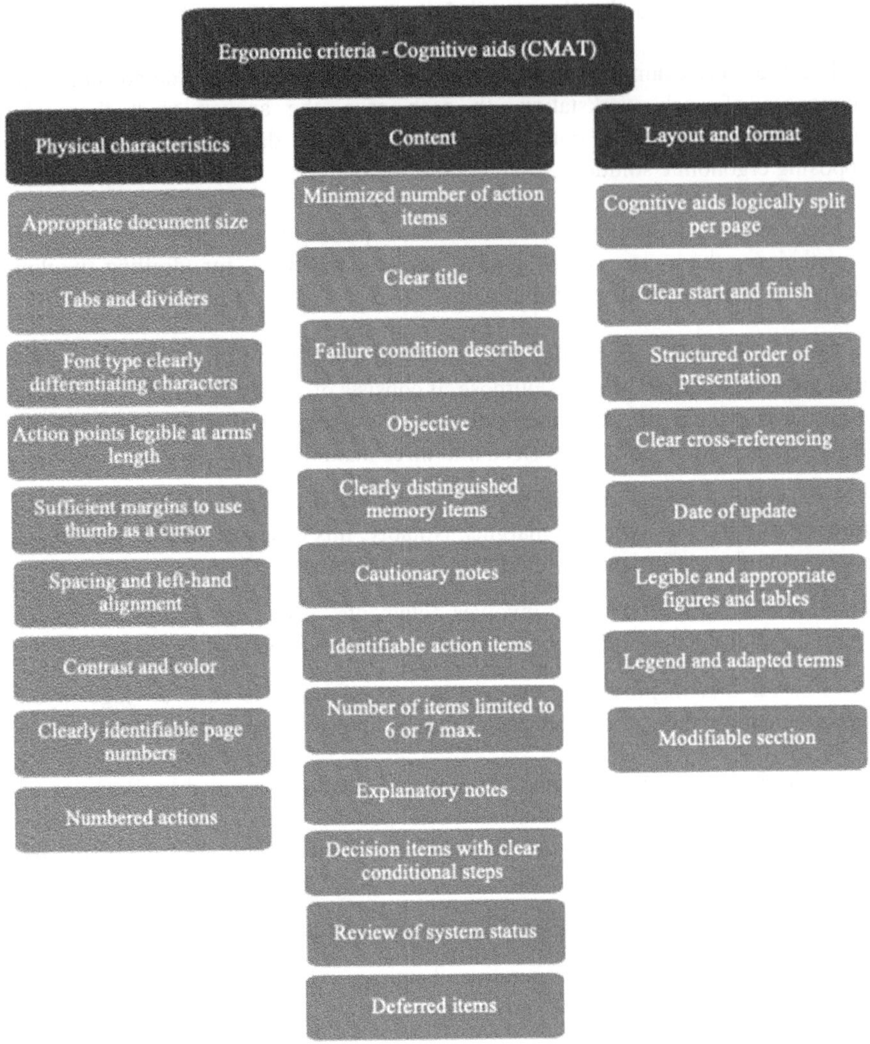

Figure 6.10. *Main elements that should compose a cognitive aid according to the CMAT design tool (criteria adapted from Evans et al. (2015) – the Association of Anaesthetists of Great Britain and Ireland). For a color version of this figure, see www.iste.co.uk/morineau/cognitive.zip*

6.3. Conclusion

A cognitive aid, such as a tape within a Turing machine, is primarily a physical object whose properties can either facilitate or burden document use. In addition to the constraints inherent in using an aid to accomplish task objectives, the prerequisite, corequisite and post-requisite phases associated with this aid should not be overlooked. Once these properties are evaluated and aligned with the constraints of the work environment, it becomes possible to consider the information to be presented on the tape. The formalism of Turing machines enables the identification of informational needs to progress within the network of mental states towards task objectives, thereby identifying strictly relevant items (as per Sperber and Wilson), known in aviation as killer items. Analyzing the work domain through an abstraction hierarchy allows for the delineation of potential paths that constitute the network of states, leading to a reconsideration of the information to be displayed on the tape. Domain analysis can also provide a list of information to be displayed at various levels of abstraction in a work assistance software, referred to as an ecological interface. Modeling operations within a work domain yields a precise model of expected tasks, serving as a benchmark against observed field conditions. Another method of designing a Turing tape is to engage experts who converge towards specifying the items to be presented in the cognitive aid (Delphi method). The designer can also rely on ergonomic criteria for document drafting.

Finally, the generic nature of the Turing machine tape allows for the conceptualization of any object as potentially constituting a cognitive aid. This is evident in examples such as the emergency reception table or through the application of the LEAN method. Here, cognitive ergonomics intersects with physical ergonomics.

However, other types of cognitive aids can be modeled using the Turing formalism. These aids do not manifest as sets of information provided by objects but rather as cognitive pathways to be followed. Such aids are more readily modeled as networks of mental states for an agent.

7

Task Analysis for Designing a Network of States

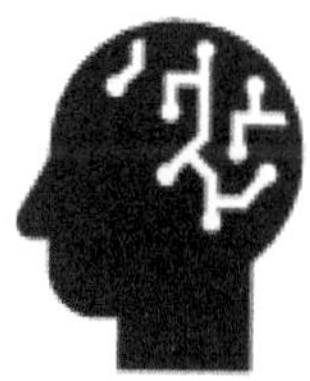

Figure 7.1. *The state transition network of a Turing machine agent*

A Turing machine's network of states accounts for a sequence of mental stages through which it is necessary to pass. The most conventional method of representing such a sequence is through an algorithm, also known as a flowchart. Operations and/or goals are logically connected in order to progress through a task until its completion. In computer science, an algorithm serves as a fundamental representation of a task designed for a computer program. However, such representations are only feasible for well-defined and generally sequential tasks, which do not typify the majority of tasks within a domain as loosely coupled as healthcare. Nevertheless, the flowchart remains a preferred mode of presenting a procedural guideline as it is grounded in the formalization of knowledge, thereby stimulating analytical thought to support reflection. Nonetheless, these flowcharts tend to be semi-formal, meaning they do not adhere to all logical requirements necessary to generate a computer program that can be operated by a machine. This semi-formal characteristic reflects the inherent challenge of fully elucidating the sequence of a task purely through logic.

For instance, the adult life support algorithm shown in Figure 7.2 includes a step inserted between two other steps, namely the action of calling 911 or a resuscitation team (Perkins et al. 2021). Formally, this representation does not adhere to the principles of algorithmics; however, in practice, it indicates the potential need to call 911 without explicitly stating the precise conditions triggering this action. Furthermore, in this algorithm, the conditions allowing progression from the heart rate evaluation step to one of the following three steps: "shockable", "return of spontaneous circulation" or "non-shockable" are also unspecified. The perception and interpretation of indicators guiding towards one of these steps (the values of physiological parameters) are left to the discretion of the rescuer. While this may be to prevent overloading the figure with information, it also implies that the algorithm, as presented, requires a certain level of expertise to be used effectively. Indeed, it serves as a description for "advanced" life support.

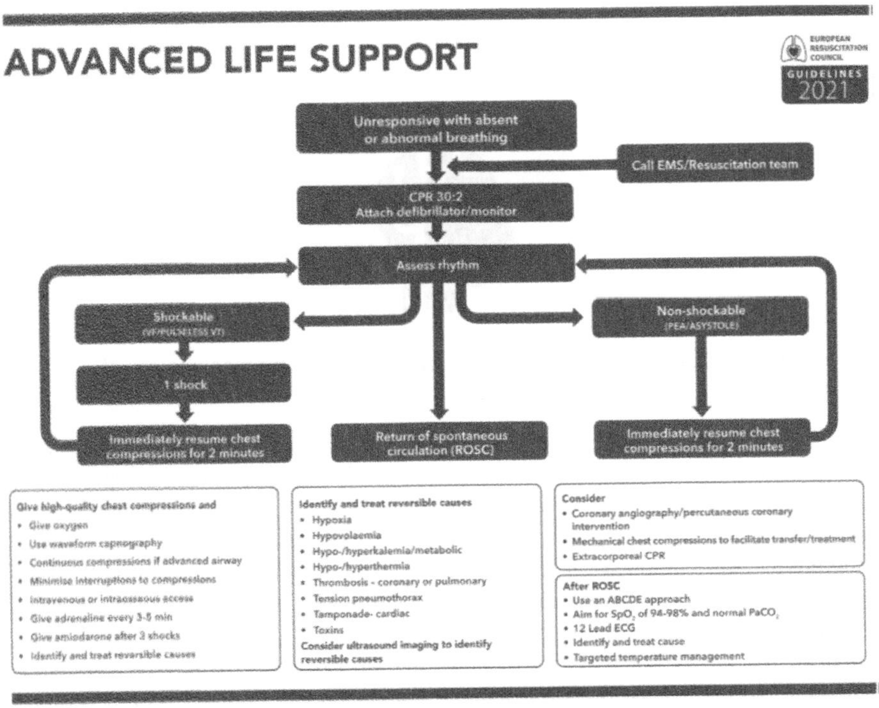

Figure 7.2. *An example of interpretable cognitive aid as a state network of a Turing machine: the advanced medical resuscitation flowchart (Perkins et al. 2021)*[1]

In accordance with the relevance standard, crafting a flowchart also involves a compromise between the effort to clarify, like an exhaustive computer algorithm

1 Available at: https://www.cprguidelines.eu/assets/guidelines/European-Resuscitation-Council-Guidelines-2021-Ad.pdf (p.126).

(exhaustiveness) and the necessity to retain a degree of implicit information left to the reader's discretion (selectivity). This implicit aspect is linked to accommodating variability in situations, which may preclude specifying certain contingent details, and avoiding information overload on the medium. Analogous to killer items on a tape, we may consider a network of strictly pertinent states (killer states). The concept suggests that these few externalized states, delineated in the cognitive aid, trigger other mental states that are well understood by the operators, who reliably access them through long-term memory. To comprehensively identify the steps of a task sequence and subsequently determine which to incorporate into the assistance mechanism, we can use the second stage of the TMTA, which involves task analysis. Indeed, *task analysis entails describing the work as a sequence of steps that must be traversed, aligning well with the logic of state networks*.

7.1. Task analysis techniques

In human factors and ergonomics, there exists a substantial array of methods for task analysis. We will discuss three of them. The first two are conceptually similar to an analysis grounded in Turing machines, while the third method merits attention due to its simplicity, making it suitable for novice analysts.

– *Navigation in the abstraction hierarchy*: building upon the use of the abstraction hierarchy to delineate a work domain, task realization can be conceptualized as navigating through the "means-to-end" relationships within this hierarchy (Miller and Vicente 1998; Morineau 2010). The various states of the network describing the task network correspond to the functions outlined in the abstraction hierarchy. This method, exemplified in the previous instance of diagnosing abdominal pain, requires a sufficiently precise analysis of the work domain to establish task sequences.

– *State Space Sketch*: another technique, not contingent upon a detailed analysis of the work domain, involves sketching the states through which it is necessary and sufficient to pass for task completion (Bernard 2020; Bernard et al. 2020). Once essential task steps are identified, their pairwise comparison elucidates how these steps may be traversed. An example of such a pairwise comparison matrix will be provided in section 7.2 on decision tree design. This method facilitates consideration of strictly pertinent states for inclusion in cognitive aids and provides a clear model of the sequence required to transition from one state to another, leading to convergence towards a Turing machine's state network.

– *Hierarchical Task Analysis (HTA) method*: a classic, straightforward method of task analysis is HTA (Annett 2004). HTA involves constructing a tree structure delineating how a task objective decomposes into sub-goals, each of which may involve further sub-subgoals or actions (see Figure 7.3). Instructions, such as iterative loops ("If sub-goal B is not achieved, perform action b1") or conditional statements ("If sub-goal B is achieved, proceed to sub-goal C"), can be integrated into an HTA tree, bringing it closer to an algorithm or Turing machine instructions.

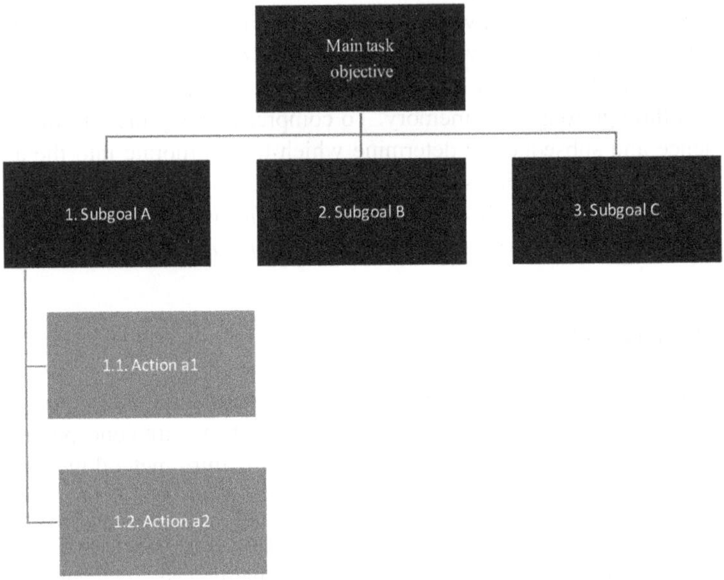

Figure 7.3. *The HTA method for modeling task achievement in goals, sub-goals and actions (adapted from Annett (2004)). For a color version of this figure, see www.iste.co.uk/morineau/cognitive.zip*

A translation of these tree structures into a state network can be carried out subsequently. We will now introduce various cognitive aids whose logic is primarily guided by defining a sequence of states to traverse.

7.2. Designing a fast and frugal tree

Previously, we explored a heuristic approach enabling quick decision-making based on a limited number of variables: fast and frugal trees. Several methods exist for designing such decision trees. The first method is the most traditional, founded on formalizing decision-making by experts who claim to base their decisions on a few fundamental parameters. Through interviews, observations and scenarios presented to experts, the objective is to elucidate the sequence of conditions for decision-making. This approach represents a classic means of extracting expertise, using accumulated expert experience to develop a shareable cognitive tool.

Another approach, also rooted in past decisions, involves conducting statistical decision analysis based on a dataset of recorded decisions. A decision tree can be automatically extracted, with the analyst determining the number of variables to consider in the tree. One example of free software for this purpose is the dtree software. The significance of this statistical data extraction method lies in its ability to reveal a decision tree that explains previous decisions, even though decision-makers are not fully conscious of it. The intuitive thinking deeply embedded in these decision trees can thus be captured by the analyst.

A third approach is to develop, in situ, a decision tree that enables quick and structured decision-making. This method will be further explored in the next section.

7.2.1. *Designing an ad hoc decision tree*

It is feasible to draw upon the state space sketch method to devise an ad hoc, fast and frugal tree, even as decision-makers grapple with a complex problem (Dormois et al. 2022). The following three steps enable the identification of relevant states necessary and sufficient for making decisions to resolve the problem. This method draws inspiration from the theory of constraints (Goldratt 1990) and encompasses the following steps:

– *Step 1: define the objective to be achieved and identify the fundamental constraints of the situation.* The objective or objectives inherent in the decision-making process must be articulated clearly. Subsequently, it involves pinpointing the critical constraints imposed by the situation, which serve as obstacles to achieving the objectives.

– *Step 2: conduct pairwise comparisons of the constraints to prioritize them.* Facilitating this comparison may involve presenting the constraints in a matrix format, facilitating a two-by-two comparison. During this process, elucidating the criteria used to prioritize one constraint over another is crucial.

– *Step 3: construct the decision tree.* Hierarchizing constraints based on their prevalence yields a tree structure that specifies the decisions necessary to satisfy this sequence of constraints. This hierarchical arrangement facilitates the development of an action plan that prioritizes actions to streamline the resolution process and enhance efficiency.

7.2.2. *A decision tree for medical-psychological reception of refugees*

This approach to decision tree design was applied, on an exploratory basis, within the context of the reception of war refugees in France by the Medical-Psychological Emergency Unit (CUMP) of Morbihan in March 2022. For the team tasked with coordinating this care, it presented an unusual intervention that imposed multiple constraints. Developing a fast and frugal tree thus became imperative to devise a modus operandi for addressing this novel situation.

The *fundamental constraints and objectives* of the situation were established: conducting debriefing interviews with the largest possible number of refugees to ensure no individuals with severe post-traumatic stress and in need of immediate psychological debriefing were overlooked. Four essential constraints pertinent to this objective were identified: interpreter availability, staff availability, refugee availability and rapid access to individuals experiencing severe post-traumatic stress. *These four constraints were then systematically compared pairwise* to establish an order of prevalence among them. Figure 7.4 shows the matrix used for this prioritization. The constraint deemed most critical among them all was interpreter availability. Without an interpreter, conducting a psychological interview is unfeasible; relying solely on automatic translation via smartphone proves inadequate. Given the limited number of CUMP stakeholders relative to the refugee population, stakeholder availability emerged as the second constraint to address. Finally, as severe trauma patients can only be reached through an initial systematic assessment of all refugees, overall refugee availability takes precedence over the accessibility of refugees with severe trauma.

	Availability of interpreters C1	Availability of care providers C2	Availability of the refugees C3	High-priority victims being reachable C4
Availability of interpreters C1		C1 > C2	C1 > C3	C1 > C4
Availability of care providers C2			C2 > C3	C2 > C4
Availability of the refugees C3				C3 > C4
High-priority victims being reachable C4				

Figure 7.4. *Matrix for pairwise comparison of variables in refugee care. "A > B" denotes: "prevalence of A over B"*

This hierarchization of variables has led to a framework for making urgent and prioritized decisions. Figure 7.5 shows the *resulting fast and frugal tree.* This decision tree facilitated the development of an action plan for the coordinators of the CUMP.

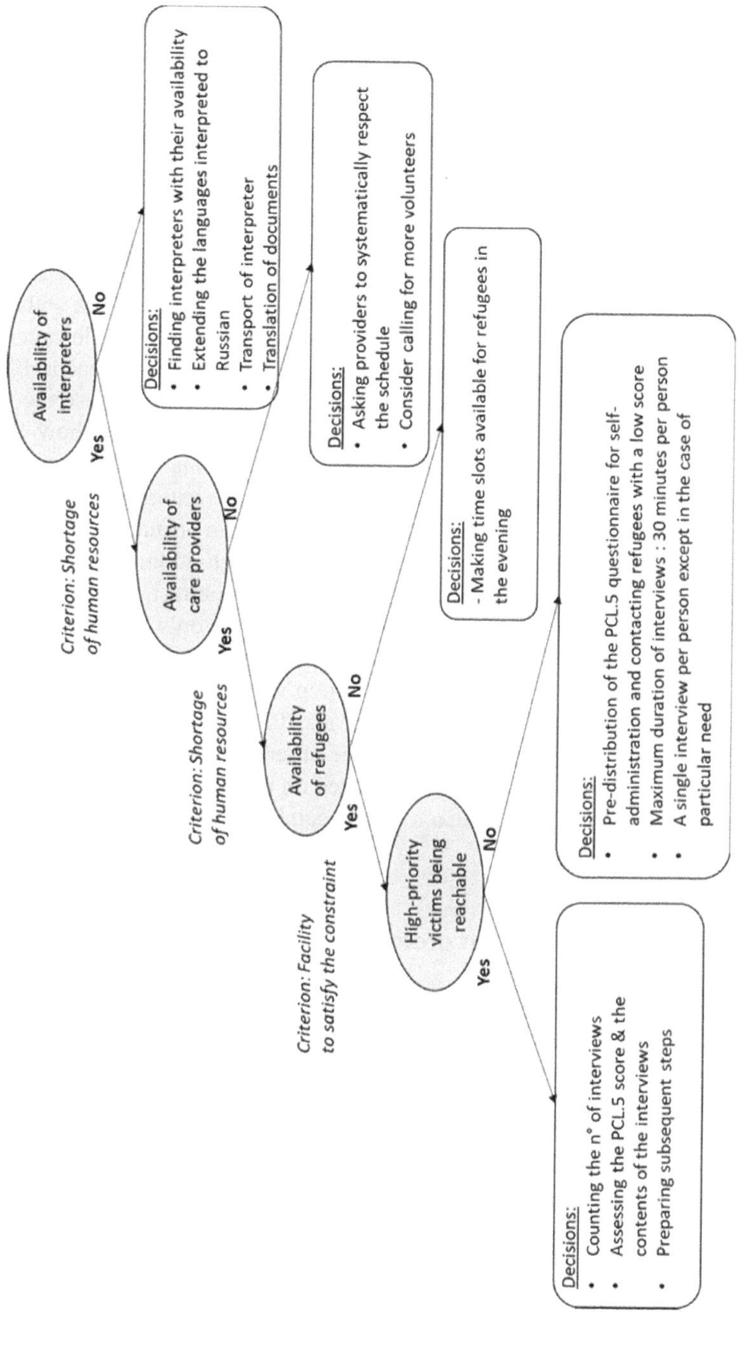

Figure 7.5. *Fast and frugal tree for the psychological care of refugees by the CUMP of Morbihan (EPSM of Saint-Avé, SAMU 56 (Dormois et al. 2022))*

Whether based on existing expert knowledge schemas, statistical analysis from a database, or ad hoc analysis of situational constraints, fast and frugal trees serve as a simple and effective decision aid, aiming for maximum relevance through a compromise between exhaustiveness and selectivity.

However, the definition of a decision tree is not without risk due to its highly selective nature. Indeed, only a limited number of variables (constraints) are considered and, furthermore, these variables are hierarchically prioritized, sometimes allowing a decision to be made before all variables are fully considered. This selectivity can lead to false negatives or false positives (Gigerenzer et al. 2022). An illustrative example of a decision tree pertains to the recruitment criteria within a company: the ultimate decision is binary (to recruit or not), and multiple criteria, hierarchically organized, may be involved. It is reported that entrepreneur Elon Musk typically recruits his staff by initially asking each candidate to describe the most challenging problem they have faced in their previous roles and how they managed to solve it. If the individual demonstrates exceptional problem-solving abilities (criterion 1), they are hired regardless of other criteria. However, a candidate may excel in this test but ultimately prove to have an unsuitable profile for the position, a risk that could have been highlighted through additional questions. This underscores the risk of producing a false positive. In contrast, Jeff Bezos, the founder of Amazon, reportedly decided to recruit a candidate only if the individual exhibited exceptional ability (criterion 1), was someone worthy of admiration (criterion 2) and contributed to raising the group's overall performance level (criterion 3) (Popomaronis 2021; Gigerenzer et al. 2022). Here, the risk of false positives is lower, but it is crucial for these three criteria to be reliable in order to avoid false negatives. The more a decision is based on a limited number of criteria, the faster and simpler it is, but it is also a bigger gamble, which, if it does not pay off, may result in a potential error.

7.3. Designing a communication protocol

By its sequential and abstract (linguistic) nature, a communication protocol can also be conceived as a series of mental states through which we must pass. For the message recipient, each mental state refers to specific information to be acquired, such as during a shift handover, an update on the current situation or a request for assistance in dealing with a challenging scenario. Similar to previous cognitive aids, the dilemma of relevance arises: whether to provide a message with comprehensive content or selective content for quick processing.

A communication protocol serves to convert an intuitive oral expression, partly implicit due to its reliance on natural language, into a structured expression based on standardized and explicit operative language, necessitating analytical thinking. To alleviate the cognitive effort required for analytical thinking, it is advisable to limit the number of items in the protocol. Using an acronym based on mnemonic devices, such as SAED for the communication protocol proposed by the French National Authority for Health (HAS 2014), facilitates easy retrieval in long-term memory by leveraging intuitive thought processes. Two levels of communication protocol implementation can be distinguished: individual-level protocols and those governing the overall organization of communications within a team.

7.3.1. *Inter-individual communication protocol*

In 2017, a US agency emphasized the importance of structured communication during medical handovers (Joint Commission 2017). This aims to prevent inaccurate, incomplete, delayed, misinterpreted or unnecessary information due to a disruptive environment or poor management of the implicit/explicit parts of the transmitted message. A well-designed information exchange protocol reduces the risk of disturbances from surrounding noise by being concise and accurate. The risk of misinterpretation is mitigated as the auditor comprehends the logic of the communication pattern. This pattern (script) serves as a framework of expectations for receiving information. With established and commonly used communication protocols, cognitive assimilation leads to automated usage. Operators intuitively apply the protocol for information exchange, representing the internalization of a psychological instrument. A communication protocol should ideally encompass two types of information: domain-specific details and peripheral information about the sender, receiver and potentially stakeholders involved.

Information regarding the work domain (patient and care) should be presented to enhance situational awareness among message receivers. Mica Endsley's concept of *situation awareness* (Endsley 1995) characterizes the mental representation of operators at work (Box 7.1).

Situation awareness encompasses:

– *the element of understanding*, rooted in previous events that provide meaningful context (the past);

– *the element of perception*, regarding access to current information (the present);

– *the projection element*, envisioning anticipated events (the future).

Box 7.1. *The concept of situation awareness (Endsley 1995)*

A communication protocol must provide information about the past, present and future concerning a patient and their required care. The Joint Commission recommendations (Joint Commission 2017) specify typical items to include:

– information about the sender, including contact details;

– pathology assessment, including severity level;

– patient summary, covering reason for admission, hospital journey and care plan;

– list of actions to be undertaken;

– specific implementation plans;

– allergy list;

– patient code;

– medication list;

– dated laboratory tests;

– dated vital signs.

Peripheral information about the receiver, sender and other potentially involved parties is as critical as patient-related data. The sender should clearly identify or locate themselves and provide a means of contact if it is a telecommunication. The message receiver must confirm correct perception and understanding of the message, with time allocated for questions and message reformulation in their own words. This is advocated by the I-PASS tool (Box 7.2).

I (Illness severity): stable, "watcher", unstable.

P (Patient summary): summary statement, events leading up to admission, hospital course, ongoing assessment, plan.

A (Action list): to-do list, timeline and ownership.

S (Situation awareness and contingency planning): know what is going on, plan for what might happen.

S (Synthesis by receiver): receiver summarizes what was heard, asks questions, restates key action/to-do items.

Box 7.2. *I-PASS communication tool (from Starmer et al. (2012))*

A study assessed the impact of the I-PASS tool in nine medical centers and among 10,740 patients. Results indicate a 30% reduction in adverse events and a 23% decrease in medical errors during its period of use (Joint Commission 2017).

7.3.2. *Protocol in teamwork*

In the context of urgently dealing with a patient, the management of oral communications within the team is a crucial factor. As previously discussed, oral expression serves as a particularly suitable psychological instrument for exchanges in emergency situations among a group of individuals directly involved in a common task. In trauma centers, optimal teamwork organization must be planned in advance to ensure multiple actions are carried out with the highest efficiency. In this regard, Hughes et al. (2014) proposed that teams in an American hospital undergo comprehensive training on communication elements deemed critical by an expert committee (see Table 7.1).

Before the patient's arrival
– Receipt of standardized and accurate patient information
– Briefing session
– Familiarization of each team member with the patient's severity level and relevant information
– Management plan by the designated leader
– Assignment of roles by the leader, especially if multiple patients are involved
During patient management
– Defined communication intervals
– Minimization of disruptions during communications (such as noise and the presence of excessive personnel)
– Awareness of the current leader
– Encouragement of open expression within the team (questions, comments)

Table 7.1. *List of communication recommendations during patient management in trauma centers (adapted from Hughes et al. (2014))*

This training has had a positive impact, as evidenced by the questionnaires completed by healthcare providers after the implementation of these recommendations. It is worth noting that the training was intensive: 15 courses, each lasting 3 hours, spread over three months. Notably, there is a recommendation for free expression within the team. Implementing this recommendation requires a non-vertical management approach that allows doctors, nurses and nursing assistants to express their opinions.

During teamwork, particularly in challenging communication situations, using the "assertions" technique can be beneficial when asking questions or making comments. This technique, as outlined by Hickey et al. (2012), involves the following steps:

– attract the attention of the message recipient by addressing them by their first name;

– express the subject of the inquiry;

– describe the status of the problem;

– propose an action to reach a decision with the interlocutor.

However, it is noted that as the complexity of the issue increases, more exchanges are required, posing the risk of diverting healthcare providers' attention from patient-related tasks. In contexts of teamwork with multiple tasks and numerous participants, clear beginnings and endings of communications are essential. At the outset of an interaction, the sender must ensure that the receiver(s) are prepared to receive the message. Upon concluding a message, the receiver should confirm their understanding, either through typical affirmations ("understood", "ok", "done") or by repeating the message. Observations of exchanges between pilots and co-pilots in aviation have shown that over time, these validation moments may become implicit (e.g. nodding, incomprehensible expression) or involve non-standardized terms, potentially leading to misunderstandings (Degani and Wiener 1990). Consequently, structured communication tends to shift from an explicit mode (system 2) to an implicit mode relying on extraverbal cues (system 1).

To ensure more reliable exchanges, it is advisable to establish a short communication loop (Härgestam et al. 2013; Bijok et al. 2022). This loop involves the transmission of an oral message from a sender to a receiver. The receiver confirms receipt of the message, allowing the sender to verify that the message has been transmitted and understood (Figure 7.6).

Upon closer examination of Figure 7.6, it becomes evident that a short communication loop resembles the establishment of a gateway between the sender and receiver of a message. It facilitates back-and-forth message exchanges between the two operators.

Once these considerations are integrated into the process of designing a cognitive aid, whether in document form or as an oral protocol, it is essential to consider how the cognitive aid will be used, i.e. the operational mode guiding its use. This operational mode can also be conceptualized as a network of states through which the user must navigate.

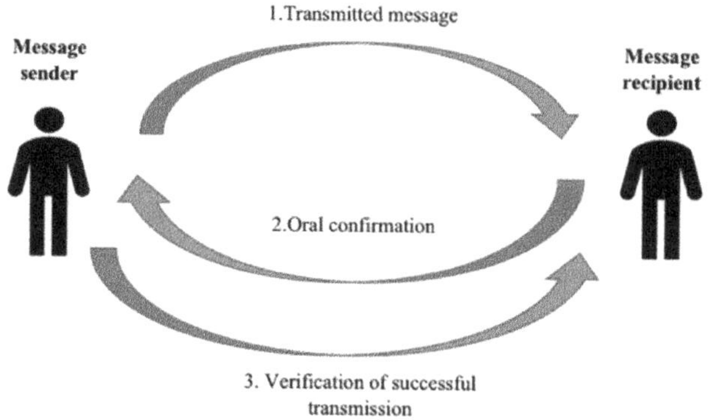

Figure 7.6. *The short communication loop ensuring the reliability of an oral message (adapted from Hārgestam et al. (2013))*

7.4. Designing the operation procedure for using a cognitive aid

Proposing an operational procedure for using a cognitive aid involves the challenge of defining a prescribed task. It involves devising a user manual for the cognitive aid. However, as previously discussed, the presence of a prescribed task implies the existence of an actual activity that, inevitably, will deviate to some extent from the prescribed task and the user manual. Cognitive aid users may not consistently adhere to the prescribed procedures. In essence, the degree of coupling between the cognitive aid and its users may be relatively loose. It is noteworthy that a cognitive aid designed to minimize the disparities between prescribed tasks and actual activities, thereby enhancing alignment between the two, can paradoxically give rise to new disparities.

In the context of a Turing machine model, the operational mode of a cognitive aid, which is the tape in this case, can be likened to the network of states through which users mentally navigate. Users engage in reading, writing and scrolling operations on the tape. These operations may pertain to concrete content such as a checklist, or abstract content like a communication protocol. In the case of abstract content, the tape serves as the users' short-term memory. For instance, when using a communication protocol, the message sender mentally adheres to the protocol activated in their short-term memory ("reading") and then communicates this protocol to the message receiver ("writing"). With this in mind, we can explore the major operational methods envisaged in cognitive aid use, followed by an examination of the effects of variability in usage observed within work contexts.

7.4.1. *Typical operating modes*

Two primary operating modes are commonly identified in the use of cognitive aids. From the perspective of a Turing machine, the first mode involves "reading" the information on the "physical" or "mental" tape (short-term memory) and then "writing" information into the environment (do). Conversely, the second mode involves "writing" (do) followed by "reading" the tape (confirming that the necessary actions have been executed).

– *Read-do mode*: in this mode, the operator reads the information provided by the cognitive aid and subsequently carries out the task. This mode mirrors the typical functionality of a user guide. The cognitive aid provides proactive guidance for the smooth execution of the activity. This *proactive mode* has the advantage of being highly efficient within a tightly coupled system. The operator is guided by the cognitive aid to perform the task reliably. It is particularly relevant for operators lacking the full expertise required for task completion or experiencing stress such that their mental state impedes their ability to initiate decisions or actions. However, a drawback is that the operator may confine their role solely to following instructions. Consequently, there is a risk of passive engagement. Moreover, in high-pressure contexts, such as those characterized by time constraints, focusing on document monitoring may divert the healthcare provider's attention away from patient examination, potentially causing them to overlook new environmental information not covered by the prescribed procedure (known as the *tunnel effect*). In this operational mode, external cognition takes precedence over internal cognition.

– *Do-confirm mode*: conversely, this operational mode involves the operator performing an action and then verifying its validity using the cognitive aid. This approach involves periodic checks at key points as the activity progresses. Activity control in this mode is *retroactively* facilitated by the cognitive aid. The primary advantage of this mode is its prioritization of operators' decisions and actions. It facilitates the functioning of a loosely coupled system. Decisions or actions are initially based on the operator's expertise and subsequently validated by the cognitive aid. This mode is well-suited to situations characterized by intense temporal pressure and involves expert operators where action takes precedence over comprehensive situation analysis, while still remaining under operator control. However, a risk associated with this mode is the *confirmation bias* that may arise. Operators may act first and then seek confirmation of their actions from the cognitive aid, potentially overlooking information that contradicts their actions. In addition, urgency may lead to prioritizing action and thus *omitting verification points*, resembling a "ballistic" action without seeking feedback on its effects. In this operational mode, internal cognition takes precedence over external cognition.

7.4.2. *Distribution of operating procedures within the team*

When considering a single user of a cognitive aid, these two operating modes, mirroring each other, are relatively straightforward to implement. However, the complexity arises when cognitive support is shared within a team. Merely having a team member use a cognitive aid individually but vocalize it aloud renders it shareable within the group, potentially leading to redundancy in item verification (cross-checking). This underscores the notion that cognition in a given situation cannot be fully understood without accounting for the cognitive system of the individual and the environment as a whole.

In the field of aeronautics, the flight crew typically consists of two pilots (sometimes three for long-haul flights). In this context, the "read-do" mode typically unfolds as follows for a checklist: Pilot A reads out the checklist items, while Pilot B carries out the instructions and communicates the effects of their actions. Conversely, in the "do-confirm" mode, Pilot A initiates actions and identifies the items being executed, while Pilots A and B collectively verify the items (cross-checking). The effectiveness of these practices hinges on the coordination between the pilots. This coordination largely depends on the leader's ability to determine whether the conditions are conducive to implementing the checklist with the co-pilot. To achieve this, the leader must anticipate their teammate's workload when using the checklist, posing the following questions (Degani and Wiener 1990):

– Is the colleague already burdened with other tasks and thus unavailable to handle the checklist?

– What are the foreseeable implications for the activity if the colleague shifts their focus to the checklist?

– What are the risks associated with postponing the checklist's implementation due to unsatisfactory current conditions?

In the medical domain, use of cognitive aids can involve more than two individuals, or even serve as a guiding or verifying tool for an entire care team (sometimes comprising five to seven individuals, particularly in pediatric emergencies). In such settings, various care processes may unfold simultaneously, including paramedical and medical care, which may involve different physicians potentially assuming leadership roles. In environments characterized by large teams, multitasking, and potentially multiple leaders, coordinating the use of cognitive aids is not straightforward. It becomes a task that must be assigned to at least one person within the team (Bernard 2020).

For a "read-do" operating method within a team, reading a cognitive aid for others immediately places the reader in a leadership role as they provide instructions. In this scenario, the senior physician, implicitly assuming a leadership position, may feel compelled to maintain this role. However, they are often already occupied with technical procedures. Hence, it is crucial to distinguish between the role of the *technical leader* guiding medical procedures and the *coordinator* responsible for providing support by disseminating information from the cognitive aid. Similarly, in a "do-confirm" procedure, a clear distinction must be made between the healthcare provider performing the action and the one verifying it, with the latter assuming the role of *supervisor*.

Once these roles are clearly defined, it does not imply that a healthcare provider cannot switch roles or simultaneously serve as both coordinator and supervisor when both modes of checklist use coexist. The choice of an operating mode can be influenced by two contextual factors.

– *The use of a cognitive aid with a shareable format* (e.g. through a large poster, screen or remote sharing in telemedicine settings), allowing anyone to assume the role of coordinator in a "read-do" process or supervisor in a "do-confirm" process.

– *Implementation of review moments* during which the entire team can collectively review actions already taken (similar to the surgical checklist). These review points facilitate monitoring of the availability of healthcare providers to use the cognitive aid.

These considerations regarding interactions with cognitive aids are valuable in prompting teams to examine their work organization and the critical issue of leadership. *Integrating cognitive aids into the cognitive system of the new agent introduces the possibility of more complex, versatile and agile relationships within the team, diverging from the conventional strictly vertical hierarchical structure.* This underscores the significance of work analysis in configuring these relationships based on observed caregiving contexts in practice.

7.4.3. *Degree of coupling in the use of cognitive aids*

A challenging aspect to address in defining the operational method of cognitive assistance in the medical field is the extent to which strict monitoring should be imposed in a given situation. This inquiry pertains to the concept of the degree of coupling between operators' activities and the tasks expected of them. Should the use of aids be enforced following an aeronautical model, characterized by a highly structured framework and strict adherence to protocols or should caregivers be empowered to determine certain aspects of use independently?

In terms of the Turing machine model, this dilemma revolves around conceptualizing cognitive aid either as a deterministic Turing machine, where the state network is predefined and must be strictly adhered to, or as a non-deterministic machine, where users have choices in situ. In the latter scenario, certain transitions between states are not predetermined, giving users discretion to navigate the variability of work contexts (such as the number of caregivers present in the team) and/or the diversity of user profiles (with experts favoring post-action verification and beginners preferring guided actions).

Within a work scenario, variations in the use of a cognitive aid by the same individual can be observed. For instance, during a simulation exercise on patient sorting at the reception of an emergency department, a participating nurse had access to a newly introduced sorting grid (the FRENCH grid) as a cognitive aid to assess the priority level of incoming patients. She had two strategies at her disposal: either directly determining the patient's sorting level in the FRENCH grid (read-do mode) or initially relying on intuition and experience to perform initial sorting, followed by validation using the FRENCH grid (do-confirm mode). During this exercise, both strategies were observed alternately among the same participants, likely influenced by their level of personal proficiency and the characteristics of the arriving patients (Régis Lorguilloux, personal communication).

7.4.4. *Attentional constraints in the use of cognitive aids*

In practical situations, using a cognitive aid with external physical support introduces a form of double tasking. The operator must simultaneously execute both their primary task and the one associated with using the cognitive aid. Notably, the more the aid's support involves prerequisites, corequisites and post-requisites, the more significant the task of using the aid becomes within the activity. This scenario can be characterized as involving:

– an *intrinsic cognitive load*, representing the mental resources allocated to performing the primary task (caregiving);

– an *extrinsic cognitive load*, stemming from the use of the cognitive aid support (Sweller et al. 2019; Puma and Tricot 2021).

To prevent interference between these tasks, it is advisable that each task draws upon cognitive resources of different natures, thereby avoiding competition for these resources. Such competition could lead to a decline in performance either in the primary task or in the handling of the cognitive aid. To describe the cognitive resources available in short-term memory (or working memory), we can reference the Wickens cube model (2008). This model delineates cognitive resources across three primary dimensions (with an additional one later added by Wickens):

– The *cognitive processing stages* specifically involved in the task: whether it involves perceptual processing, short-term memory retention or a behavioral response.

– *Information encoding*: whether it involves spatial, verbal or action-related encoding (speech, manual control).

– The *primary sensory modalities* engaged in information processing: whether the task involves auditory or visual modalities.

– To these three dimensions, Wickens later added a distinction within visual perception, differentiating between *foveal and peripheral vision* engagement in the task.

If two tasks draw upon the same resources across these dimensions of the cube, the risk of interference between them increases. Conversely, if two simultaneous tasks do not share the same cognitive resources, increasing the difficulty of one task will not affect the performance of the other task (*principle of difficulty insensitivity*).

For instance, consider the use of GPS while driving. If the GPS guidance relies solely on an on-screen display, there is a risk of interference between tracking the trajectory while driving and attending to the GPS information. Alternatively, if the GPS provides information through text-to-speech, it reduces the shared cognitive resources. Indeed, these two tasks share identical resources on the three dimensions: in terms of cognitive processing stage (perceptual task of information collection), information coding (spatial coding) and sensory modality (visual perception). However, if the GPS provides information through a text-to-speech synthesis, this reduces the number of shared resources. Moreover, it should be noted that if the visual display of the GPS is placed peripherally in the driver's field of view, this reduces interference with the foveal vision task primarily involved in driving (fourth dimension of the Wickens cube). Therefore, from a cognitive analysis of the operators' main task in the context of using a cognitive aid, it is possible, thanks to the Wickens cube, to consider the interaction modes to be defined for the cognitive aid so that it does not interfere with the main task.

7.4.5. Recommendations for designing a network of states

Monitoring the stages of a network of states also imposes attentional constraints on the user. Several ergonomic recommendations for graphically presenting a network of states (flowchart) to reduce attentional effort can be suggested.

– States can be represented as simple points or as larger graphical entities (e.g. circles, rectangles, diamonds). The more intricate the graphics, the more potential for informational noise they introduce. Therefore, graphical simplicity is preferred.

– Sequential relationships can be depicted through an ordered sequence of items horizontally, vertically or even transversely (ascending or descending sequences). Items can be separated by spaces, lines, commas or indicated by transitions with lines or arrows. Symbols that change shape over time can also represent sequences, such as the temporal sequence displayed by a digital stopwatch.

– The meanings of each symbol used in the graph must be clear, including the shape, color and significance of shapes representing states (e.g. circles, rectangles) and transitions between stages (arrows).

– A legend may be necessary if the symbols are multifold, have complex meanings or are potentially polysemous.

– Avoid overloading the graph with information and avoid creating crossings in the paths between states. Reading a flowchart requires perceptual effort due to the need to follow an ocular trajectory within the network.

– Avoid creating paths in the graph that lead the operator to adopt a passive "agentic" state, where they follow the path without considering their actions. This can occur when the graph is segmented, showing only the current step to be processed. In such cases, the user loses the overall view of the task's progress, along with the global awareness needed to make sense of their actions and anticipate future tasks.

7.4.6. *Operating modes observed in real-world activity*

The use of cognitive aids in context inevitably varies from what was planned. This phenomenon, conventionally described in ergonomics, is associated with the variability and scalability of the environment, on the one hand, and the variability and scalability of user profiles, on the other hand. Examples in aeronautics show the intervention of these two factors in use (Degani and Wiener 1990).

7.4.6.1. *Environmental factor*

The use of cognitive support must occur at the appropriate moment and within the right context to ensure that the individuals involved are mentally available. The presence of pre-existing mental workload or distractors may interfere with this availability. An aviation accident, such as that of Northwest Airlines Flight 255 in 1987, was caused by the failure to use a taxi checklist on the runway within the first one or two minutes as planned, due to several interruptions (including new weather information). Consequently, the contextual cues necessary to initiate use of the checklist had disappeared, leading to its hasty application thereafter and the omission of a critical item required for aircraft takeoff.

7.4.6.2. *Individual factor*

Repetition associated with the routine use of an aid can bring about significant changes in use. It has been observed in aircraft cockpits that pilots streamline the flow of checklist items by consolidating several items into one – a cognitive process known as *chunking*. While this accelerates task completion, it also introduces the risk of haste in processing the items within each chunk. Cognitive automation in the use of aids poses inherent risks. Interviews with pilots reveal instances in which they mistakenly believed they had verified the normal status of checklist items when they had not. Processing information through automated scripts tends to heavily prioritize expected values for each item based on typical observations, *effectively turning these commonly observed values into default standards*. This cognitive bias, rooted in intuitive thinking, can be exacerbated by adverse working conditions such as stress, temporal pressure, high workload, fatigue and noise (Staal 2004). In addition, there is a trend towards increasingly implicit communication over time. It is worth noting that this automation of interactions with aids is not necessarily negative; it can reflect a growing mutual understanding resulting from team stability. The shift towards implicit communication streamlines work processes and reduces ambient noise associated with explicit verbal messages.

7.4.6.3. *"Individual–environment" interaction*

Cognitive automation in the use of assistance can lead to an optimization point in the use of cognitive resources, both external and internal. For the same activated knowledge schemas, part of it will rely on external resources, while the other part will draw upon mental resources preserved by the operator. A *script* can be understood as a knowledge network primarily comprising a node used to initiate the script, on the one hand, and a set of reinforced connections between different knowledge nodes, activated by this initiation, on the other hand. In this structure, initiation relies on external cues serving as resources to trigger the script, while knowledge with strong connections belongs to the internal resources of the individual. This routine mode of operation with distributed cognition is evident in the use of cognitive aids. A compelling illustration is seen in the example of a pilot observed reciting the contents of a checklist, while merely placing his hand on the paper of this checklist, without consulting its contents (Degani and Wiener 1990). The mere sensorimotor pointing to a physical cue enables access to the content, once again highlighting the strong links between the environment and the individual in an entire cognitive system in which cognition is distributed.

The phenomenon of initiation through the situation of memorized knowledge is termed in psychology the *context-dependent memory effect*. Farnsworth (1934), a psychologist, proposed to students of similar levels teachings that occurred either in the same room as the final exam or in a different room. The results show a slightly higher performance among students who took their exam in the same room as the course. Godden and Baddeley (1975), on the contrary, tasked their participants, members of a diving club, with memorizing and then recalling a list of words either on the beach or underwater (about 7 meters deep). The results indicate that performance drops only when participants change the context between the memorization phase and the recall phase. The context of encoding information serves as a natural and unconscious cognitive aid for memory retrieval, even in challenging contexts such as underwater.

An experiment we conducted suggests that this context-dependent memory effect occurs simply by having in one's visual field the document whose content was memorized during recall. This finding corroborates the previous observation made in the cockpit (Morineau et al. 2005). This context-dependent memory effect underscores the importance of evaluating a new aid in the context of its use, whether real or simulated. Evaluation constitutes a critical phase of the design process.

7.4.7. *Evaluation of cognitive aid usage*

For several years now, the process of designing any technical device has been viewed as a "design-evaluation" cycle. An iterative evaluation of mock-ups, prototypes and final products is necessary to avoid critical errors. Since device evaluation is a domain in itself, it is impractical to delve into methodological details (evaluation protocols, objective and subjective methods, data processing) here. Readers interested in further exploration of this aspect are referred to methodology manuals, particularly in cognitive psychology, ergonomics and statistics in the humanities and medical sciences. Similarly, we will not discuss statistical techniques here for ensuring the validity and reliability of document content.

Regarding cognitive aids, three main evaluation modalities can be distinguished: experimental evaluation, in situ evaluation and systemic evaluation. As part of a comprehensive evaluation process, these three steps can be carried out in sequence.

7.4.7.1. *Experimental evaluation*

The development of simulation environments in healthcare, recreating care settings, now allows for not only professional training but also the evaluation of new cognitive aids in a realistic context. By constructing situations that replicate the cognitive system of a caregiver, it becomes possible to measure behaviors following an experimental protocol logic (manipulated sources of variation, measured variables, controlled conditions). The availability of mobile video devices facilitates the transposition of simulations into professionals' premises, thereby bringing observed situations closer to real-world contexts. Rapid software mock-ups also enable the evaluation of multiple versions of the device under scrutiny.

Beyond faithfully replicating working conditions, simulation allows for the creation of "surreal" situations, meaning scenarios that artificially modify certain parameters to study their impact. For instance, breaking down a medical procedure into sub-steps, each simulated separately, is feasible. In addition, functionally impossible configurations can be tested to emphasize crucial aspects of the situation. For example, caregivers can be blindfolded during a simulation to underscore the importance of other sensory cues or the guidance of action through voice cues (Morgan Jaffrelot, personal communication).

7.4.7.2. *Evaluation of cognitive aids in real-world settings*

One of the challenges in simulation experimentation is the frequent absence of longitudinal measurement. Without this dimension, it is challenging to observe the processes of acquisition and appropriation as they unfold over time. To address this, it is preferable to transition to monitoring the use of the device in actual work settings. Monitoring the introduction of a new device involves observations, interviews and online questionnaires, ensuring anonymity. This type of evaluation greatly benefits from pre- and post-implementation measures to assess the impact on work. This methodological framework requires anticipation of the evaluation to gather data on activity before the device is deployed in the field.

7.4.7.3. *Systemic evaluation*

On a broader scale and over a longer period, studying the impact on the functioning of a service or workstation allows for a comprehensive understanding of the consequences of introducing cognitive aids into the cognitive system. Research using this approach has demonstrated that the effects of an aid extend beyond the mere document or protocol itself.

For instance, Bosk et al. (2009) observe that the increase in safety attributed to a checklist is not solely due to the physical document but also encompasses the broader implications of its presence in the work system during its design phase. The researchers tracked the implementation of a checklist in the intensive care units of Michigan hospitals in 2006 to mitigate the risks associated with catheter placement. Prior to checklist implementation, each hospital appointed medical and paramedical leaders to be responsible for the project. These leaders regularly engaged with the teams, addressed their concerns and provided solutions collaboratively. In addition, the leaders received safety training and then imparted knowledge to the teams, maintaining ongoing communication with them. The teams collected data on catheter-related infections, and caregivers contributed insights on managing infectious risks. In this context, the checklist represents just one component of a broader strategy that fostered team acculturation to risk, skill enhancement and consideration of their work dynamics and challenges. The authors argue against the notion that a checklist alone is a cost-effective and straightforward solution for significantly reducing risks in hospitals. Instead, they emphasize that a cognitive aid must be integrated into a comprehensive organizational approach to safety, requiring constructive managerial dynamics within the institution.

The other dimension upon which the integration of a cognitive aid into a work system is developed concerns the indirect effects that this device will produce on the activity, beyond the expected direct effects. For example, the implementation of the WHO Surgical Checklist in the operating room may have altered the operational flow in certain hospitals. The pause required in care to verify the checklist items became an additional step in the process, leading to discretization of the continuous activity flow. The necessity for team members to verbally confirm a set of information led caregivers to communicate more than usual. According to Barnes et al. (2015), the effectiveness of the surgical checklist primarily lies in its function as a platform for discussing risks, specifics of planned surgery and individual concerns, giving voice to each member of the operating room team, reducing hierarchical verticality and facilitating the detection of safety issues (Imhof 2019). From the perspective of the operating protocol, the checklist compelled some hospitals to alter their operational procedures, especially in terms of the administration of antibiotics. The checklist promotes the administration of antibiotics in the operating room rather than in the preoperative room, where delays may impact drug efficacy. In addition, previously overlooked physiological measures, such as airway assessment and oximetry, have been instituted.

The WHO Surgical Safety Checklist implementation manual indicates that the checklist is not merely a document but also an organizational mode of operation. It notes that "a single person must be made responsible for performing the safety checks on the list. This designated Checklist coordinator will often be a circulating nurse, but it can be any clinician participating in the operation". Anticipating the potential drawbacks of assigning a single person to manage the checklist, the guide states:

> [a] possible disadvantage of having a single person lead the Checklist is that an antagonistic relationship might be established with other operating team members. The Checklist coordinator can and should prevent the team from progressing to the next phase of the operation until each step is satisfactorily addressed, but in doing so may alienate or irritate other team members. Therefore, hospitals must carefully consider which staff member is most suitable for this role. As mentioned, for many institutions this will be a circulating nurse, but any clinician can coordinate the Checklist process (WHO 2009b).

These indications demonstrate that a checklist or any other form of cognitive aid cannot be introduced into a work system without anticipating the actual effects it will have on the organization of the overall system.

7.5. Conclusion

By conceptualizing a cognitive aid as akin to a Turing machine, a comprehensive framework for analyzing work can be established, allowing for the consideration of assistance requirements. This methodological framework, known as TMTA, comprising both domain analysis and task analysis, facilitates the characterization of aids based on whether they function as informational supports (analogous to the tape of a Turing machine) or procedures facilitating task progression (analogous to the state network of the machine). This model emphasizes the importance of identifying relevant information (killer items) facilitating task transitions and relevant states in decision-making or task execution. Once the pre-introduction work analysis of the new cognitive aid is completed, it becomes imperative to replicate this analysis at the level of interaction between the aid and its prospective users. Here again, the Turing machine model is applicable: the user navigates through mental states, while using the tape that constitutes the cognitive aid, either a physical tape or merely symbolic in short-term memory when recalling a given protocol, such as a communication protocol. In this context, the use of the cognitive aid should be seen as a secondary task compared to the main task, which is the caregiving task. This dual-task situation leads to a more or less extensive sharing of identical cognitive resources between the two tasks, which can result in interference in the activity.

However, the study cannot conclude at this point. Given that caregiving work is typically a team effort, it is crucial to consider the interaction modalities between different caregivers and the cognitive aid. The role of the cognitive aid may involve directing decisions and actions or serving as a downstream verification tool. Moreover, the presence of multiple human and artificial agents (the cognitive aide) necessitates considering their coordination as a distinct task. This involves assigning one or more conductor roles to teammates in a relatively permanent way, such as technical leader, coordinator or supervisor roles. These considerations allow for envisioning cognitive aid use and defining evaluation scenarios to test the hypotheses derived from this projection. Nonetheless, it is essential to recognize that cognitive aid alone is not sufficient or fully representative of its potential benefits. It constitutes part of a new equilibrium introduced to the overall work system. This new systemic equilibrium, in its various facets, must mitigate potential side effects to enhance patient safety and caregiver job satisfaction.

Table 7.2 provides a summary of tools for work analysis aimed at designing a cognitive aid.

Device to be designed	**Turing machine**	**Model components**	**Analysis and specification tools**
Checklist, to-do list, software, etc.	Tape	Information content Relevant items	Domain analysis (abstraction hierarchy, Delphi method, etc.)
		Appearance Material form Manipulations of the physical support	Ergonomic criteria Prerequisites, corequisites, post-requisites. LEAN method
Flowchart, decision tree, communication protocol, etc.	Agent's mental state network	Objectives, steps, constraints Relevant states Relationships between states	Task analysis (navigation in the abstraction hierarchy, state space sketches, HTA, etc.) Recommendations for designing a state network
Modes of interaction with the cognitive aid	Agent's mental state network	Operational modes	*Read-do, do-confirm* *Cross-checking*
		Main (care) and secondary (cognitive aid) tasks	Assigned roles in the team (supervisor, coordinator, leader) Wickens' cube: involved cognitive resources

Table 7.2. *Summary of elements for designing a cognitive aid based on the Turing machine model*

Conclusion

The observation of a pilot in a cockpit, placing his hand on a checklist and reciting its contents from memory during an aircraft check, provides valuable insights into the potential benefits of cognitive assistance. This example underscores the various functions of a gateway, a role that a cognitive aid must fulfill to constitute genuine assistance.

As a conduit between external and internal knowledge, this simple act of referencing the checklist represents an optimized allocation of cognitive resources between the environment and the individual. Although the implementation of cognitive aid depends on the environment, the operator has assimilated its contents to the extent that they can be recalled from memory. The pilot remained actively engaged throughout the prior use of the checklist, avoiding a passive stance that might have resulted in the loss of associated skills during the verification phase. Instead, upon externalizing the verification procedure through the provision of the checklist, an internalization process occurred, demonstrating the checklist's effectiveness as a psychological instrument. Nonetheless, the physical presence of the cognitive aid remains essential to serve as a priming cue.

In this example, the integration of intuitive and analytical knowledge is also prominent. While the checklist, with its structured nature and exhaustiveness, prompts analytical thinking, the internalization of its use transforms it into an automated script embedded in intuitive thought.

Similarly, regarding the alignment between the prescribed task and actual activity, strict adherence to the checklist by the pilot ensures a robust link between the procedure and its execution. However, the pilot's development of an original strategy to carry out this procedure demonstrates the ability to exercise degrees of freedom and use an unconventional operating mode, diverging from expectations.

While no innovation is introduced in terms of the checklist's content, innovation exists in its usage method.

Determine the need for the checklist	
Identify the goal and the recipient of the checklist	
Develop content using the following:	Broad spectrum of peer-reviewed literature Expert judgment Consensus among relevant opinion leaders Multidisciplinary input Consideration of current practices
Design must consider:	Context for the checklist Readability Proper categorization of information Structure of checkpoints Limited use of images Appropriate use of color Avoid jargon – use common terminology Flow of real-time user activities Clinical state of mind
Pilot test – validation in simulated clinical environment is a must	
Review with appropriate multidisciplinary representation	
Obtain approval from appropriate regulatory authorities as required, prior to implementation in the clinical environment	
Develop an education plan to properly train users	
Frequent review of evidence-based checklist content	

Table C.1. *Steps for designing a checklist (from Hales et al. (2008))*

This example of checklist use epitomizes an ideal scenario for integrating a cognitive aid within an "individual–environment" cognitive system, achieving equilibrium in knowledge activation and distribution. In this setup, the device functions solely as a gateway between the individual and the environment, without needing to manage the cognitive resources' transfer between points. Physically, this gateway aligns with the pilot's extended hand towards the document. Here, the concept of knowledge indexing is apt: the pilot indicates a set of knowledge with their index finger. However, achieving such symbiosis is challenging in multi-operator work systems with high situational variability, as seen in healthcare. To approach this, a rigorous design framework is essential. Hales et al. (2008) offer a series of steps detailed in Table C.1 for developing a checklist, which can be generalized to other types of cognitive aid.

To refine the initial two stages involving the analysis of needs and identification of goals and recipients, we can incorporate inquiries regarding the concept of a cognitive gateway.

– *What primary external resources need to be provided*: resources for verification, decision-making, action execution and memorization tasks?

– *How can cognitive resources within the system be made easily accessible, reliable and trustworthy* in their effectiveness towards achieving the specified objectives?

– *In what ways will the cognitive aid serve as a psychological instrument* for its users, fostering active engagement and providing assistance that enhances the overall capacities of the cognitive system?

– *Is there a preference for routing analytical or intuitive resources?*

– *Should there be a greater emphasis on explicating knowledge or reducing the degree of explanation* to facilitate intuitive decision-making and representations in uncertain environments, and which type of cognitive aid would be most suitable for this purpose?

– *What directives and prescriptions need to be conveyed and how should degrees of freedom be preserved in actual activities* to enable effective loose coupling, thereby ensuring system resilience?

Subsequent design process steps can benefit from the Turing machine model in specifying cognitive aid characteristics. Depending on the type of cognitive aid, the following questions may arise.

For a cognitive aid resembling a tape:

– *What are the physical characteristics* (affordances) of the tape?

– *What actions are required to fulfill prerequisites, corequisites, and post-requisites*, and how can they be minimized?

– Given the task procedure associated with the cognitive aid, *are the squares and symbols on the tape essential and sufficient* to trigger progression within the network of mental states?

– *How can information (symbols) be presented for easy readability and understanding*?

For a cognitive aid structured as a network of mental states:

– *How can a flowchart be formalized* to ensure easy comprehension without inducing operator passivity?

– *Considering the multitude of variables influencing decisions, how can they be prioritized* into a fast and frugal tree?

– *What operational mode should be adopted for using the aid*: read-do/do-confirm, individually or collectively, and how should roles be distributed?

In the design of a tape or a network of mental states to pass through, the definition of necessary and sufficient resources emerges as a pivotal element of the design process. It is noteworthy that this criterion guided Alan Turing's work in developing his machine model. This criterion also evokes the concept of frugality, which pertains to the use of essential and sufficient technological resources to design a device that relies minimally on vulnerable technologies in crisis situations (such as cyberattacks, power outages, etc.).

Resilience holds a significance in the healthcare domain that may surpass that of mere performance in care. Reflecting on the cognitive aids we discussed, many were notably frugal: floor strips to designate individuals' positions around the patient's bed; an organized table for managing records; a paper sheet for initial patient contact; a frugal decision tree; briefing points within teams. Frugal innovation offers an optimized approach on all fronts (ergonomic, economic, technological) to enhance both working conditions and patient safety. Recalling William of Ockham's "razor" or principle of parsimony, which suggests limiting the sophistication of thoughts in intellectual productions: the simplest solution often proves to be the best.

However, beyond the design of cognitive aids, examining a work situation in these terms provides an insightful understanding of the operator, particularly the healthcare professional. A caregiver's role extends beyond their work tasks; they are part of a cognitive system heavily influenced by the external environment upon which their cognition relies or falters when this environment is inadequate. Moreover, a significant part of their expertise resides in tacit knowledge schemas, some of which may remain inaccessible to consciousness in their entirety. These methodological principles underscore the necessity of not being limited to interviewing individuals or to questionnaires in order to understand work situations, but to analyze work by using diverse information gathering techniques, including observation and experimentation, guided by a comprehensive framework such as cognitive work analysis (CWA), to fully comprehend cognitive systems in work contexts.

In this book, we have primarily discussed cognitive aids for professionals, particularly those in the healthcare field. However, given the increasing complexity of the world and the abundance of circulating information, the concept of cognitive aid holds promise for everyone in their daily lives. As noted by researcher Stanovich (2018), a leading figure in psychology focusing on analytical and intuitive cognitive systems, problem-solving situations with inherent traps, often presented to students in laboratory settings, are not merely artificial constructs. Instead, they reflect the growing prevalence of real-world scenarios designed to induce cognitive biases in decision-making. Advertising, marketing and social media platforms, along with their influencers, create environments that discourage analytical thinking, favoring quick reactions over reasoned judgment. Despite the proliferation of information, Herbert Simon's concept of bounded rationality remains pertinent. Also, amidst this information overload, brief messages and provocative imagery prompt instinctive responses, leaving little time for inhibition and reasoned analysis. For Stanovich, this process corresponds to the transition from a socio-technical environment that was initially considered somewhat benign, to an environment that proves to be rather hostile. One way to move towards a benevolent environment could be to view information systems as full-fledged cognitive aids, facilitating activation of the mental resources needed to inhibit primary reactions and to facilitate access to complex reasoning. In this approach, a computer or smartphone would not be a mere commonplace tool for buying, selling, messaging, influencing others or processing information, but would fully assume the role of a psychological instrument capable of bridging the gap between the environment and the individual, between their various cognitive resources.

However, to accept this cognitive assistance function, we must be able to have a certain degree of confidence in this device and acknowledge that our mind is not self-sufficient. This implies tolerating the idea that we are dependent on the external environment; this environment can take the form of artificial intelligence. It is necessary to admit that cognition is fundamentally distributed and that cognitive aids constitute an ordinary way for humans to reason actively.

In refining the ergonomics of cognitive aids, the ultimate goal would be to achieve the optimal balance exemplified by a pilot merely pointing to a checklist to access its content. This involves designing cognitive aids that serve as priming cues for knowledge without passively storing it. Finally, an ideal cognitive aid is one that would resemble books that show up on the shelves of a library, or yellowed photos on display on a piece of furniture, in other words an indexing device. Perhaps the best cognitive aid is the one that is never consulted, but whose unique presence ensures access to knowledge.

References

Abelson, R.P. (1981). Psychological status of the script concept. *Am. Psychol.*, 36(7), 715.

ANACT (2008). *Pénibilité au travail. Une approche par les processus d'usure et les itinéraires professionnels*. Éditions ANACT, Paris.

Anderson, J.R. (1992). Automaticity and the ACT theory. *Am. J. Psychol.*, 105(2), 165–180.

Annett, J. (2004). Hierarchical task analysis (HTA). In *Handbook of Human Factors and Ergonomics Methods*, Stanton, N.A., Hedge, A., Brookhuis, K., Salas, E., Hendrick, H.W. (eds). CRC Press, Boca Raton.

Ashby, W.R. (1958). Requisite variety and its implications for the control of complex systems. *Cybernetica*, 1(2), 83–99.

Audétat, M.-C. (2012). L'identification et la remédiation des difficultés de raisonnement clinique en médecine (État des pratiques, recherche d'outils et processus pour soutenir les cliniciens enseignants). PhD Thesis, Université de Montréal, Montréal.

Audétat, M.-C., Laurin, S., Dory, V., Charlin, B., Nenda, M. (2017). Diagnostic et prise en charge des difficultés de raisonnement clinique. Guide AMEE no. 11. *Pédagogie Médicale*, 18(3), 139–149.

Baddeley, A. (1992). Working memory. *Science*, 255(5044), 556–559.

Barnes, C., Berry, W., Edmondson, L., Childers, A.K. (2015). Safe surgery checklist implementation guide [Online]. Available at: https://www.ariadnelabs.org/wp-content/uploads/2018/08/safe_surgery_implementation_guide__092515.012216_.pdf [Accessed 5 March 2023].

Bartlett, F. (1932). *Remembering*. Cambridge University Press, New York.

Basso Werle, N., Saurin, T.A., Soliman, M. (2019). Collaborative use of slack resources as a support to resilience: Study of a maternity ward. In *Working Across Boundaries, Resilient Health Care*, Braithwaite, J., Hollnagel, E., Hunte, G.S. (eds). CRC Press, Boca Raton.

Benoît, C. and Passerat-Boulade, C. (2020). *Manager dans le secteur sanitaire et médico-social*. GERESO Éditions, Le Mans.

Berenholtz, S.M., Pronovost, P.J., Lipsett, P.A., Hobson, D., Earsing, K., Farley, J.E., Milanovich, S., Garrett-Mayer, E., Winters, B.D., Rubin, H.R. et al. (2004). Eliminating catheter-related bloodstream infections in the intensive care unit. *Crit. Care Med.*, 32(10), 2014–2020.

Bernard, C.I. (2020). Analyse de l'activité de soignants médicaux et paramédicaux sur simulateur haute-fidélité lors de simulations d'urgence, en vue de la conception d'un environnement de soins ergonomique. PhD Thesis, Université de Bretagne Sud, Vannes.

Bernard, C.I., Morineau, T., Thierry, S. (2020). The degrees of freedom problem: How to guide trajectories with the dynamic safety model to assist activity in loosely coupled work systems. *Saf. Sci.*, 127, 104712.

Bernard, C.I., Thierry, S., Morineau, T. (2021). Turing machine task analysis: Specifying emergency assistance functions for a telemedicine system. *Cogn. Technol. Work*, 23(4), 771–781.

Bijok, B., Jaulin, F., Picard, J., Michelet, D., Fuzier, R., Arzalier-Daret, S., Basquin, C., Blanié, A., Chauveau, L., Cros, J. et al. (2022). Facteurs humains en situations critiques. Recommandations de pratiques professionnelles [Online]. Available at: https://sfar.org/download/recommandations-de-pratiques-professionnelles-facteurs-humains-ensituation-de-crise/ [Accessed 6 March 2023].

Blanié, A., Gorse, S., Kurrek, M., de Saint Maurice, G., Trouiller, P., Ehooman, F., Benhamou, D. (2018). Enquête sur la connaissance et l'utilisation des aides cognitives de crise en anesthésie réanimation en France en 2017. In *Congrès de la SoFraSimS*, Caen.

Bokhari, M.B., Patel, C.B., Ramos-Valadez, D.I., Ragupathi, M., Haas, E.M. (2011). Learning curve for robotic-assisted laparoscopic colorectal surgery. *Surg. Endosc.*, 25(3), 855–860.

Bosk, C.L., Dixon-Woods, M., Goeschel, C.A., Pronovost, P.J. (2009). Reality check for checklists. *Lancet*, 374(9688), 444–445.

Boulanger, B., Broche-Valence, C., Perron, J.-B., Lorguilloux, R., Morineau, T. (2021). Concevoir un assistant digital pour la prise en charge des urgences vitales. In *29e colloque national des centres d'enseignement en soins d'urgence*.

Boyne, W.J. (2013). The checklist. *Air Force Mag.*, 96(8), 52–56.

Brangier, E. and Barcenilla, J. (2001). Comment évaluer et améliorer la qualité des aides textuelles fournies aux opérateurs ? In *Signalétique : conception, validation, usages*, de Lavalette, B., Doré, J., Tijus, C. (eds). Lavoisier, Paris, 93–107.

Broom, M.A., Capek, A.L., Carachi, P., Akeroyd, M.A., Hilditch, G. (2011). Critical phase distractions in anaesthesia and the sterile cockpit concept. *Anaesthesia*, 66(3), 175–179.

Burns, C.M. and Hajdukiewicz, J. (2017). *Ecological Interface Design*. CRC Press, Boca Raton.

Carroll, E. (1988). The role of tacit knowledge in problem solving in the clinical setting. *Nurse Educ. Today*, 8(3), 140–147.

Chaparro, A., Keebler, J.R., Lazzara, E.H., Diamond, A. (2019). Checklists: A review of their origins, benefits, and current uses as a cognitive aid in medicine. *Ergon. Des.*, 27(2), 21–26.

Chapelain, P., Morineau, T., Gautier, C. (2015). Effects of communication on the performance of nursing students during the simulation of an emergency situation. *J. Adv. Nurs.*, 71(11), 2650–2660.

Chrimes, N. (2016). The Vortex: A universal "high-acuity implementation tool" for emergency airway management. *Br. J. Anaesth.*, 117(1), i20–i27.

Clark, A. and Chalmers D. (1998). The extended mind. *Analysis*, 58(1), 7–19.

Cleeremans, A., Destrebecqz, A., Boyer, M. (1998). Implicit learning: News from the front. *Trends Cogn. Sci.*, 2(10), 406–416.

Coldewey, B., Diruf, A., Röhrig, R., Lipprandt, M. (2022). Causes of use errors in ventilation devices – Systematic review. *Appl. Ergon.*, 98, 103544.

Conein, B. (2004). Cognition distribuée, groupe social et technologie cognitive. *Réseaux*, 2, 53–79.

Cook, R. and Rasmussen, J. (2005). "Going solid": A model of system dynamics and consequences for patient safety. *BMJ Qual. Saf.*, 14(2), 130–134.

Croskerry, P. (2003). The importance of cognitive errors in diagnosis and strategies to minimize them. *Acad. Med.*, 78(8), 775–780.

Croskerry, P. (2009). Clinical cognition and diagnostic error: Applications of a dual process model of reasoning. *Adv. Health Sci. Educ.*, 14, 27–35.

Croskerry, P., Singhal, G., Mamede, S. (2013). Cognitive debiasing 2: Impediments to and strategies for change. *BMJ Qual. Saf.*, 22(2), ii65–ii72.

Cvach, M. (2012). Monitor alarm fatigue: An integrative review. *Biomed. Instrum.*, 46(4), 268–277.

Debouck, F., Rieger, É., Petit, H., Noël, G., Ravinet, L. (2012). Méthode Orion® : analyse systémique simple et efficace des événements cliniques et des précurseurs survenant en pratique médicale hospitalière. *Cancer/Radiother.*, 16(3), 201–208.

Degani, A. and Wiener, E.L. (1990). Human factors of flight-deck checklists: The normal checklist. Contractor Report (CR), NASA [Online]. Available at: https://ntrs.nasa.gov/api/citations/19910017830/downloads/19910017830.pdf.

DeMiguel, V., Garlappi, L., Uppal, R. (2009). Optimal versus naive diversification: How inefficient is the 1/N portfolio strategy? *Rev. Financ. Stud.*, 22, 1915–1953.

Desnoyer, A., Blanc, A.L., Pourcher, V., Besson, M., Fonzo-Christe, C., Desmeules, J., Perrier, A., Bonnabry, P., Samer, C., Guignard, B. (2017). PIM-Check: Development of an international prescription-screening checklist designed by a Delphi method for internal medicine patients. *BMJ Open*, 7(7), e016070.

Dormois, I., Cainjo, T., Raimbault, C., Morineau, T. (2022). L'arbre de décision rapide et frugal pour organiser l'urgence médico-psychologique : application à l'accueil des réfugiés ukrainiens. In *3e Journées de la FTSLU*, Caen.

DREES (2009). Enquête nationale sur la survenue d'événements indésirables graves associés aux soins en 2009, ENEIS 2 [Online]. Available at: solidarites-sante.gouv.fr.

Dryver, E., Forberg, J.L., Segerstad, C.H., Dupont, W.D., Bergenfelz, A., Ekelund, U. (2021). Medical crisis checklists in the emergency department: A simulation-based multi-institutional randomised controlled trial. *BMJ Qual. Saf.*, 30(9), 697–705.

Endsley, M.R. (1995). Measurement of situation awareness in dynamic systems. *Hum. Factors*, 37(1), 65–84.

Evans, D., McCahon, R., Barley, M., Norris, A., Khajuria, A., Moppett, I. (2015). Cognitive aids in medicine assessment tool (CMAT): Preliminary validation of a novel tool for the assessment of emergency cognitive aids. *Anaesthesia*, 70(8), 922–932.

Falzon, P. (1987). Langages opératifs et compréhension opérative. *Trav. Hum.*, 50(3), 281–286.

Farnsworth, P.R. (1934). Examinations in familiar and unfamiliar surroundings. *J. Soc. Psychol.*, 128–129.

Fitts, P.M. (1951). *Human Engineering for an Effective air Navigation and Traffic Control System*. National Research Council, Washington.

Flach, J.M. (2012). Complexity: Learning to muddle through. *Cogn. Technol. Work*, 14(3), 187–197.

Fletcher, G., Flin, R., McGeorge, P., Glavin, R., Maran, N., Patey, R. (2003). Anaesthetists' non-technical skills (ANTS): Evaluation of a behavioural marker system. *Br. J. Anaesth.*, 90(5), 580–588.

Flin, R. (2013). Non-technical skills for anaesthetists, surgeons and scrub practitioners (ANTS, NOTSS and SPLINTS). *The Healthcare Foundation*, 1–9.

Friedrich, J. (2012). L'idée d'instrument psychologique chez Vygotski. *Riv. ital. filos. linguaggio*, 6(2), 189–201.

Fuchs, A., Haller, M., Riva, T., Nabecker, S., Greif, R., Berger-Estilita, J. (2021). Translation and application of guidelines into clinical practice: A colour-coded difficult airway trolley. *Trends Anaesth. Crit.*, 40, 46–54.

Gaba, D.M., Howard, S.K., Small, S.D. (1995). Situation awareness in anesthesiology. *Hum. Factors*, 37(1), 20–31.

Gagliardi, A.R., Straus, S.E., Shojania, K.G., Urbach, D.R. (2014). Multiple interacting factors influence adherence, and outcomes associated with surgical safety checklists: A qualitative study. *PLoS One*, 9(9), e108585.

Ganier, F. (2018). *Comprendre la documentation technique*. Presses Universitaires de France, Paris.

Garcia-Retamero, R. and Galesic, M. (2010). Who profits from visual aids: Overcoming challenges in people's understanding of risks. *Soc. Sci. Med.*, 70(7), 1019–1025.

Gaver, W.W. (1991). Technology affordances. In *Proceedings of CH'91 (New Orleans)*, 28 April–2 May. ACM, New York [Online]. Available at: https://www.lri.fr/~mbl/Stanford/CS477/papers/Gaver-CHI1991.pdf.

Georges, P.M. and Samson, J. (2012). *Gérer un hôpital, un pôle*. Sauramps Medical, Paris.

Gibson, J.J. (1979). *The Ecological Approach to Visual Perception*. Erlbaum, Hillsdale.

Gigerenzer, G. and Gaissmaier, W. (2011). Heuristic decision making. *Annu. Rev. Psychol.*, 62, 451–482 [Online]. Available at: https://economics.northwestern.edu/docs/events/nemmers/2018/gigerenzer2.pdf.

Gigerenzer, G. and Kurzenhaeuser, S. (2005). Fast and frugal heuristics in medical decision making. In *Science and Medicine in Dialogue*, Bibacc, R., Laird, J.D., Noller, K.L., Valsiner, J. (eds). Praeger, Wesport.

Gigerenzer, G., Reb, J., Luan, S. (2022). Smart heuristics for individuals, teams, and organizations. *Annu. Rev. Organ. Psychol.*, 9, 171–198.

Gobet, F. (1998). Memory for the meaningless: How chunks help. In *Proceedings of the 20th Meeting of the Cognitive Science Society*, 398–403 [Online]. Available at: https://citeseerx.ist.psu.edu/document?repid=rep1&type=pdf&doi=098993cfb25200e266c9ec08bf349e83da229a6f.

Godden, D.R. and Baddeley, A.D. (1975). Context-dependent memory in two natural environments: On land and underwater. *Br. J. Psychol.*, 66(3), 325–331.

Goldratt, E.M. (1990). *Theory of Constraints*. North River Press, Croton on Hudson.

Goody, J. (1979). *La domestication de la pensée sauvage*. Éditions de Minuit, Paris.

Granger, B. (2022). *Excel m'a tuer. L'hôpital fracassé*. Odile Jacob, Paris.

Hafenbrädl, S., Waeger, D., Marewski, J.N., Gigerenzer, G. (2016). Applied decision making with fast-and-frugal heuristics. *J. Appl. Res. Mem. Cog.*, 5(2), 215–231.

Hajdukiewicz, J. and Burns, C. (2004). Strategies for bridging the gap between analysis and design for ecological interface design. In *Proceedings of the Human Factors and Ergonomics Society Annual Meeting*, 48(3), 479–483.

Hales, B., Terblanche, M., Fowler, R., Sibbald, W. (2008). Development of medical checklists for improved quality of patient care. *Int. J. Qual. Health Care*, 20(1), 22–30.

Hams, S.P. (2000). A gut feeling? Intuition and critical care nursing. *Intensive Crit. Care Nurs.*, 16(5), 310–318.

Hancock, P.A. and Weaver, J.L. (2005). On time distortion under stress. *Theor. Issues Ergon.*, 6(2), 193–211.

Hansten, R. (2003). Streamline change-of-shift report. *Nurs. Manage.*, 34(8), 58–59.

Härgestam, M., Lindkvist, M., Brulin, C., Jacobsson, M., Hultin, M. (2013). Communication in interdisciplinary teams: Exploring closed-loop communication during in situ trauma team training. *BMJ Open*, 3, e003525.

HAS (2014). Saed : un guide pour faciliter la communication entre professionnels de santé [Online]. Available at: https://www.has-sante.fr/jcms/c_1776178/fr/saed-un-guide-pour-faciliter-la-communication-entre-professionnels-de-sante [Accessed 13 March 2023].

HAS (2019). La simulation en santé [Online]. Available at: https://www.has-sante.fr/jcms/c_930641/fr/simulation-en-sante [Accessed 8 March 2023].

Haynes, A.B., Weiser, T.C., Berry, W.R., Lipsitz, S.R., Breizat, A-H S., Dellinger, E.P., Herbosa, T., Joseph S., Kibatala, P.L., Lapitan M.C.M. et al. (2009). A surgical safety checklist to reduce morbidity and mortality in a global population. *N. Engl. J. Med.*, 360, 491–499.

Hickey, P., Connor, J.A., Trainor, B., Brostoff, M., Blum, R., Jenkins, K., Stuart-Shor, E. (2012). Implementation of an organization-wide standardized communication initiative. *J. Healthc. Commun.*, 5(1), 32–39.

Hollnagel, E. (2011). The requisite variety of risk assessment: Catching up with nature. Plenary Lecture, ESREL 2011, 18–22 September, Troyes [Online]. Available at: https://static1.squarespace.com/static/53b78765e4b0949940758017/t/57180e3c2fe131333b8bf2ea/1461194316142/_Requisite+Variety+of+Risk+Assessment-+Catching+up+with+nature+Hollnagel.pdf.

Hollnagel, E. (2018). *Safety-I and Safety-II: The Past and Future of Safety Management.* CRC Press, Boca Raton.

Houdé, O. (1995). *Rationalité, développement et inhibition : un nouveau cadre d'analyse.* Feni, Paris.

Howard, S.K., Gaba, D.M., Fish, K.J., Yang, G., Sarnquist, F.H. (1992). Anesthesia crisis resource management training: Teaching anesthesiologists to handle critical incidents. *Aviat. Space Environ. Med.*, 63(9), 763–770.

Hughes, K.M., Benenson, R.S., Krichten, A.E., Clancy, K.D., Ryan, J.P., Hammond, C. (2014). A crew resource management program tailored to trauma resuscitation improves team behavior and communication. *J. Am. Coll. Surg.*, 219(3), 545–551.

Hutchins, E. (1995). *Cognition in the Wild.* MIT Press, Cambridge.

Idal Sznelwar, L., Lancman, S., Wu, M.J., Alvarinho, E. (1983). Analyse du travail dans un service de nettoyage hospitalier : contributions de l'analyse ergonomique du travail et d'un groupe de réflexion inspire de l'approche de la psychodynamique du travail. In *38e congrès de la SELF*, Paris, 423–430.

IEA (n.d.). Définition de l'ergonomie [Online]. Available at: https://iea.cc/about/what-is-ergonomics [Accessed 8 March 2023].

Imhof, A. (2019). En quoi la check-list chirurgicale est-elle bien plus qu'une liste à cocher [Online]. Available at: https://www.securitedespatients.ch/ [Accessed 6 March 2023].

Jaffrelot, M. and Pelaccia, T. (2016). La simulation en santé : principes, outils, impacts et implications pour la formation des enseignants. *Recherche & Formation*, 82, 17–30.

Jaffrelot, M., Boet, S., Cioccio, A.D., Michinov, E., Chiniara, G. (2013). Simulation et gestion de crise. *Réanimation*, 22(6), 569–576.

Jaffrelot, M., Weiss, A., Derrien, P., Borraccia, I., Vidailhet, P. (2016). Préparer et animer une séance de simulation. In *Comment (mieux) former et évaluer les étudiants en médecine et en sciences de la santé*, Pelaccia, T. (ed.). De Boeck, Louvain-la-Neuve.

Javadi, A.H., Emo, B., Howard, L.R., Zisch, F.E., Yu, Y., Knight, R., Pinelo Silva, J., Spiers, H.J. (2017). Hippocampal and prefrontal processing of network topology to simulate the future. *Nat. Commun.*, 8(1), 14652.

Jenkins, B. (2014). Cognitive aids: Time for a change? *Anaesthesia*, 69(7), 660–664.

Joint Commission (2017). Inadequate hand-off communication. *Sentinel Event Alert*, 58(1), 6.

Joulé, R.V. and Beauvois, J.L. (2002). *Petit traité de manipulation à l'usage des honnêtes gens*. Presses universitaires de Grenoble, Grenoble.

Kaempf, G.L., Klein, G., Thordsen, M.L., Wolf, S. (1996). Decision making in complex naval command-and-control environments. *Hum. Fact.*, 38(2), 220–231.

Kahneman, D. (1973). *Attention and Effort*. Prentice-Hall, Englewood Cliffs.

Kahneman, D. (2011). *Thinking, Fast and Slow*. Farrar, Straus and Giroux, New York.

Kahneman, D., Sibony, O., Sunstein, C.R. (2021). *Noise: A Flaw in Human Judgment*. HarperCollins, London.

Kaufman, E.L., Lord, M.W., Reese, T.W., Volkmann, J. (1949). The discrimination of visual number. *Am. J. Psychol.*, 62(4), 498–525.

Kendra, J. and Wachtendorf, T. (2003). Creativity in emergency response to the World Trade Center disaster. *Account Post Disas. Res.*, 1997, 121–146.

Klein, G. (1993). A recognition primed decision (RDP) model of rapid decision making. In *Decision Making in Action: Models and Methods*, Klein, G., Oransu, J., Calderwood, R., Zsambok, C. (eds). Ablex, New York.

Klein, G. (2008). Naturalistic decision making. *Hum. Factors*, 50(3), 456–460.

Kohn, K.T., Corrigan, J.M., Donaldson, M.S. (1999). *To Err Is Human: Building a Safer Health System*. National Academy Press, Washington.

Landucci, F. and Lamperti, M. (2021). A pandemic of cognitive bias. *Intensive Care Med.*, 47(5), 636–637.

Langlois, M. and Ploquin, F. (2016). *Médecin du RAID*. Albin Michel, Paris.

Lasater, K. (2011). Clinical judgment: The last frontier for evaluation. *Nurse Educ. Pract.*, 11(2), 86–92.

Lauber, J. (1979). Resource management on the flight deck. Background and statement of the problem. In *Proceedings of NASA/Industry Workshop*, San Francisco, 3–16.

Leape, L.L., Lawthers, A.G., Brennan, T.A., Johnson, W.G. (1993). Preventing medical injury. *QRB Qual. Rev. Bull.*, 19(5), 144–149.

Leplat, J. (1977). Les facteurs déterminant la charge de travail. Rapport introductif. *Trav. Hum.*, 40(2), 195–202.

Leplat, J. and Hoc, J.M. (1983). Tâche et activité dans l'analyse psychologique des situations. *Cahiers de psychologie cognitive*, 3(1), 49–63.

Loyd, G.E., Lake, C.L., Greenberg, R.B. (eds) (2004). *Practical Health Care Simulations.* Hanley & Belfus, Philadelphia.

Luan, S., Schooler, L.J., Gigerenzer, G. (2011). A signal-detection analysis of fast-and-frugal trees. *Psychol. Rev.*, 118(2), 316–338.

Martignon, L., Katsikopoulos, K.V., Woike, J.K. (2008). Categorization with limited resources: A family of simple heuristics. *J. Math. Psychol.*, 52(6), 352–361.

Maudsley, G. and Strivens, J. (2000). Promoting professional knowledge, experiential learning and critical thinking for medical students. *Med. Educ.*, 34(7), 535–544.

McGeorge, N., Hegde, S., Berg, R.L., Guarrera-Schick, T.K., LaVergne, D.T., Casucci, S.N., Hettinger, A.Z., Clark, L.N., Lin, L, Fairbanks, R.J. et al. (2015). Assessment of innovative emergency department information displays in a clinical simulation center. *J. Cogn. Eng. Decis.*, 9(4), 329–346.

Mendonca, D.J. and Al Wallace, W. (2007). A cognitive model of improvisation in emergency management. *IEEE Trans. Syst. Man Cybern. A Syst. Hum.*, 37(4), 547–561.

Michel, P., Quenon, J.-L., Daucourt, V., Burdet, S., Hoarau, D., Klich, A., Pourin, C., Rabilloud, M., Colin, C. (2022). Incidence des événements indésirables graves associés aux soins dans les établissements de santé (ENEIS 3) : quelle évolution dix ans après ? *BEH*, 13, 229–237.

Miller, G.A. (1956). The magical number seven, plus or minus two: Some limits on our capacity for processing information. *Psychol. Rev.*, 63(2), 81.

Miller, C.A. and Vicente, K.J. (1998). Toward an integration of task- and work domain analysis techniques for human-computer interface design. In *Proceedings of the Human Factors and Ergonomics Society Annual Meeting*, 42(3), 336–340.

Ministère des Solidarités et de la Santé (2019). Guide d'aide à la préparation et à la gestion des tensions hospitalières et des situations sanitaires exceptionnelles [Online]. Available at: https://solidarites-sante.gouv.fr/IMG/pdf/guide_situation_sanitaire_exceptionnelle.pdf [Accessed 6 March 2023].

Minvielle, E. (2018). *Le patient et le système. En quête d'une organisation sur mesure.* Seli Arslan, Paris.

Mol, A. (2008). *The Logic of Care. Health and the Problem of Patient Choice.* Routledge, London.

Morineau, T. (2010). La méthode TMTA d'analyse écologique de la tâche et son application à une tâche praxique. *Trav. Hum.*, 73(2), 97–122.

Morineau, T. (2011). Turing machine task analysis: A method for modelling affordances in the design process. *J. Eng. Des.*, 4(1), 58–70.

Morineau, T. and Djenidi-Delfour, M. (2023). Modèle SHELL : une cartographie pour analyser son espace de travail. In *Facteurs humains en santé – Analyse et gestion du risque*, Fuzier, R. and Jaulin, F. (eds). Arnette, Paris.

Morineau, T. and Flach, J.M. (2019). The heuristic version of cognitive work analysis: A first application to medical emergency situations. *Appl. Ergon.*, 79, 98–106.

Morineau, T., Blanche, C., Tobin, L., Guéguen, N. (2005). The emergence of the contextual role of the e-book in cognitive processes through an ecological and functional analysis. *Int. J. Hum. Comput.*, 62(3), 329–348.

Morineau, T., Morandi, X., Le Moëllic, N., Diabira, S., Riffaud, L., Haegelen, C., Hénaux, P.-L., Jannin, P. (2009a). Decision making during preoperative surgical planning. *Hum. Factors*, 51(1), 67–77.

Morineau, T., Frénod, E., Blanche, C., Tobin, L. (2009b). Turing machine as an ecological model for task analysis. *Theor. Issues Ergon.*, 10(6), 511–529.

Morineau, T., Morandi, X., Le Moëllic, N., Jannin, P. (2013). A cognitive engineering framework for the specification of information requirements in medical imaging: Application in image-guided neurosurgery. *Int. J. Comput. Assist. Radiol. Surg.*, 8(2), 291–300.

Morineau, T., Chapelain, P., Quinio, P. (2016). Task management skills and their deficiencies during care delivery in simulated medical emergency situation: A classification. *Intensive Crit. Care Nurs.*, 34, 42–50.

Morineau, T., Chapelain, P., Le Courtois, M., Le Gac, J.M. (2017). Fields of promoted actions for facilitating multitasking activity during a medical emergency. *BMJ Simul. Technol. Enhanc. Learn.*, 3(2), 70–72.

Morineau, T., Djenidi-Delfour, M., Arnault, F. (2021). Designing affordance-based procedures using heuristic cognitive work analysis: Application to triage in an emergency department. *J. Cogn. Eng. Decis.*, 15(4), 198–212.

Nibbelink, C.W. and Reed, P.G. (2019). Deriving the practice-primed decision model from a naturalistic decision-making perspective for acute care nursing research. *Appl. Nurs. Res.*, 46, 20–23.

Norman, D.A. (1988). *The Psychology of Everyday Things*. Basic Books, New York.

Norman, D.A. and Shallice, T. (1980). Attention to action: Willed and automatic control of behavior. In *Consciousness and Self-Regulation*, Davidson, R.J., Schwartz, G.E., Shapiro, D. (eds). Springer, Boston, MA [Online]. Available at: http://wexler.free.fr/library/files/norman%20%28%29%20attention%20to%20action.%20willed%20and%20automatic%20control%20of%20behavior.pdf.

Oléron, P. (1977). *Le raisonnement.* Que sais-je ? Presses Universitaires de France, Paris.

ORSAS (2009). La méthode Delphi. Documentary record. ORSAS, Lorraine.

O'Sullivan, E. and Schofield, S. (2018). Cognitive bias in clinical medicine. *J. R. Coll. Physicians Edinb.*, 48(3), 225–231.

Parent, F. and Jouquan, J. (2013). *Penser la formation des professionnels de la santé. Une perspective intégrative.* De Boeck, Brussels.

Paul, R.W. and Heaslip, P. (1995). Critical thinking and intuitive nursing practice. *J. Adv. Nurs.*, 22(1), 40–47.

Pelaccia, T. (2016a). Vers une perspective sociocognitiviste de l'étude du raisonnement clinique pour mieux capter l'expertise. Un éclairage particulier à partir de l'étude du raisonnement en médecine d'urgence. *Pédagogie Médicale*, 17(4), 255–260.

Pelaccia, T. (2016b). *Comment (mieux) former et évaluer les étudiants en médecine et en sciences de la santé ?* De Boeck Supérieur, Louvain-la-Neuve.

Peran, D., Kodet, J., Pekara, J., Mala, L., Truhlar, A., Cmorej, P.C., Lauridsen, K.G., Sari, F., Sykora, R. (2020). ABCDE cognitive aid tool in patient assessment – Development and validation in a multicenter pilot simulation study. *BMC Emerg. Med.*, 20(1), 1–8.

Perkins, G.D., Graesner, J.T., Semeraro, F. et al. (2021). European resuscitation council guidelines 2021: Executive summary. *Resuscitation*, 161, 1–60.

Piaget, J. (1937). *La construction du réel chez l'enfant.* Delachaux, Neuchatel.

Piché, D. (2005). *Intuition et abstraction. Textes de Guillaume d'Ockham*. Vrin, Paris.

Popomaronis, T. (2021). Elon Musk asks this question at every interview to spot a liar – Why science says it actually works. *CNBC Make It* [Online]. Available at: https://www.cnbc.com/2021/01/26/elon-musk-favorite-job-interview-question-to-ask-to-spot-a-liar-science-says-it-actually-works.html [Accessed 8 March 2023].

Pronovost, P., Needham, D., Berenholtz, S., Sinopoli, D., Chu, H., Cosgrove, S., Sexton, B., Hyzy, R., Welsh, R., Roth, G. et al. (2006). An intervention to decrease catheter-related bloodstream infections in the ICU. *The New England Journal of Medicine*, 355(26), 2725–2732.

Puma, S. and Tricot, A. (2021). Prendre en compte la mémoire de travail lors de la conception de situations d'apprentissage scolaire. *Analyse neuropsychologique des apprentissages chez l'enfant*, 171, 217–225.

Rasmussen, J. (1985). The role of hierarchical knowledge representation in decision making and system management. *IEEE Trans. Syst. Man Cybern. A Syst. Hum.*, 2, 234–243.

Rasmussen, J. (1986). *Information Processing and Human-Machine Interaction. An Approach to Cognitive Engineering*. North-Holland, Amsterdam.

Rasmussen, J. (1990). The role of error in organizing behaviour. *Ergonomics*, 33(10/11), 1185–1199.

Reber, A.S. (1989). Implicit learning and tacit knowledge. *J. Exp. Psychol. Gen.*, 118(3), 219.

Reuchlin, M. (1978). Processus vicariants et différences individuelles. *J. Psychol.*, 2, 133–145.

Richard, J.F. (1990). *Les activités mentales : comprendre, raisonner, trouver des solutions*. Armand Colin, Paris.

Rieul, G. (2019). Développement et évaluation d'une application multiplateforme d'organisation et de partage de la connaissance médicale pour les internes d'Anesthésie-Réanimation. Medicine Thesis, Université Rennes 1, Rennes.

Rivenc, F. (1989). *Introduction à la logique*. Payot, Paris.

Roehr, C.C., Schmölzer, G.M., Thio, M., Dawson, J.A., Dold, S.K., Schmalisch, G., Davis, P.G. (2014). How ABBA may help improve neonatal resuscitation training: Auditory prompts to enable coordination of manual inflations and chest compressions. *J. Paediatr. Child Health*, 50(6), 444–448.

Russ, S., Rout, S., Caris, J., Mansell, J., Davies, R., Mayer, E., Moorthy, K., Darzi, A., Vincent, C., Sevdalis, N. (2015). Measuring variation in use of the WHO surgical safety checklist in the operating room: A multicenter prospective cross-sectional study. *J. Am. Coll. Surg.*, 220(1), 1–11.

SafeTeam Academy (2020). Newsletter April 2020 [Online]. Available at: https://www.anesthesiasafetynetwork.com/pdf/fr/2020-04-ASN15-fr.pdf [Accessed 6 March 2023].

Scarpina, F. and Tagini, S. (2017). The stroop color and word test. *Front. Psychol.*, 8(557).

Schneuwly, B. (1987). Les capacités humaines sont des constructions sociales. Essai sur la théorie de Vygotsky. *Eur. J. Psychol. Educ.*, 1(4), 5–16.

Schreiber, M. (2010). The psySTART rapid mental health triage and incident management system. PhD Thesis, University of California, Los Angeles.

Schreiber, M., Yin, R., Omaish, M., Broderick, J.E. (2014). Snapshot from Superstorm Sandy: American Red Cross mental health risk surveillance in lower New York State. *Ann. Emerg. Med.*, 64(1), 59–65.

Sebillotte, S. (1995). Methodology guide to task analysis with the goal of extracting relevant characteristics for human-computer interfaces. *Int. J. Hum-Comput. Int.*, 7(4), 341–363.

SFAR (n.d.). Aides cognitives [Online]. Available at: https://sfar.org/download-category/aides-cognitives/page/4/ [Accessed 7 March 2023].

Simon, H.A. (1945). *Administrative Behavior: A Study of Decision-Making Processes in Administrative Organization*. The Free Press, New York.

Simpson, E. and Courtney, M. (2002). Critical thinking in nursing education: Literature review. *Int. J. Nurs. Pract.*, 8(2), 89–98.

Sperber, D. and Wilson, D. (1989) *La pertinence. Cognition et communication*. Éditions de Minuit, Paris.

Staal, M.A. (2004). Stress, cognition, and human performance: A literature review and conceptual framework. NASA-TM-2004-212824 [Online]. Available at: https://core.ac.uk/download/pdf/10517392.pdf.

Stanovich, K.E. (2018). Miserliness in human cognition: The interaction of detection, override and mindware. *Think. Reason.*, 24(4), 423–444.

Starck, C., Thierry, S., Bernard, C.I., Morineau, T., Jaulin, F., Chapelain, P., Komorowski, M. (2020). Tracheal intubation in microgravity: A simulation study comparing direct laryngoscopy and videolaryngoscopy. *Br. J. Anaesth.*, 125(1), e47–e53.

Starmer, A.J., Spector, N.D., Srivastava, R., Allen, A.D., Landrigan, C.P., Sectish, T.C., I-PASS study group (2012). I-pass, a mnemonic to standardize verbal handoffs. *Pediatrics*, 129(2), 201–204.

Suchman, L.A. (1987). *Plans and Situated Actions: The Problem of Human-Machine Communication*. Cambridge University Press, Cambridge.

Sweller, J. and Cooper, G. (1985). The use of worked examples as a substitute for problem solving in learning algebra. *Cogn. Instr.*, 2, 59–89.

Sweller, J., Van Merriënboer, J., Paas, F. (2019). Cognitive architecture and instructional design: 20 years later. *Educ. Psychol. Rev.*, 31, 261–292.

Truog, R.D., Mitchell, C., Daley, G.Q. (2020). The toughest triage – Allocating ventilators in a pandemic. *N. Engl. J. Med.*, 382(21), 1973–1975.

Turing, A.M. (1936). On computable numbers, with an application to the Entscheidungsproblem. *J. Math.*, 58(345/363), 5.

Tversky, A. and Kahneman, D. (1974). Judgment under uncertainty: Heuristics and biases: Biases in judgments reveal some heuristics of thinking under uncertainty. *Science*, 185(4157), 1124–1131.

Van den Bruel, A., Thompson, M., Buntinx, F., Mant, D. (2012). Clinicians' gut feeling about serious infections in children: Observational study. *Brit. Med. J.*, 345, e6144.

Vanpee, D., Frenay, M., Godin, V., Bédard, D. (2009). Ce que la perspective de l'apprentissage et de l'enseignement contextualisés authentiques peut apporter pour optimaliser la qualité pédagogique des stages d'externat. *Pédagogie Médicale*, 10(4), 253–266.

Venkateswaran, S., Nahmens, I., Ikuma, L. (2013). Improving healthcare warehouse operations through 5S. *IISE Trans. Healthc. Syst. Eng.*, 3(4), 240–253.

Vicente, K.J. (1999). *Cognitive Work Analysis: Toward Safe, Productive, and Healthy Computer-Based Work*. CRC Press, Boca Raton.

Vicente, K.J. and Rasmussen, J. (1992). Ecological interface design: Theoretical foundations. *IEEE Trans. Syst. Man Cybern. A Syst. Hum.*, 22(4), 589–606.

Vortex Approach (n.d.). The Vortex approach to airway management [Online]. Available at: http://vortexapproach.org/ [Accessed 7 March 2023].

Vygotsky, L. (2012). *Thought and Language*. MIT Press, Cambridge.

Wells, A.J. (2004). *Cognitive Science and the Turing Machine: An Ecological Perspective*. Springer, Berlin, Heidelberg.

WHO (2009a). WHO surgical safety checklist [Online]. Available at: https://www.who.int/teams/integrated-health-services/patient-safety/research/safe-surgery/tool-and-resources.

WHO (2009b). Implementation manual – WHO surgical safety checklist 2009: Safe surgery saves lives [Online]. Available at: https://iris.who.int/handle/10665/44186.

Wickens, C.D. (2008). Multiple resources and mental workload. *Hum. Factors*, 50(3), 449–455.

Zelano, N. (2014). Pénibilité au travail : élaboration d'un guide diagnostique méthodologique. PhD Thesis, Université Toulouse III, Toulouse.

Index

C, D

E, F

G, H

I, J

T, U

V, W

Other titles from

ISTE

in

Health Engineering and Society

2024

SARAZIN Marianne
Artificial Intelligence in Health
(Technological Prospects and Social Applications Set – Volume 7)

2023

BEYALA Laure
Digital Therapy: The New Age of Healthcare
(Technological Prospects and Social Applications Set – Volume 6)

CORROY Laurence, CHAUZAL-LARGUIER Christelle
Patients, Caregivers and Doctors: Devices, Issues and Representations
(Communication and Health Set – Volume 1)

SOMMER Pascal, DEBRET Romain
The Elasticity of Life: From Tissues to Humans

2022

ASSAILLY Jean-Pascal
Child Psychology: Developments in Knowledge and Theoretical Models
(Health and Patients Set – Volume 3)

CHAABANE Sondès, COUSEIN Etienne, WIESER Philippe
Healthcare Systems: Challenges and Opportunities

PAGANELLI Céline, CLAVIER Viviane
Information Practices and Knowledge in Health
(Health and Patients Set – Volume 5)

SALGUES Bruno, BARNOUIN Jacques
The Covid-19 Crisis: From a Question of an Epidemic to a Societal Questioning
(Health and Patients Set – Volume 4)

2021

BÉRANGER Jérôme
Societal Responsibility of Artificial Intelligence: Towards an Ethical and Eco-responsible AI
(Technological Prospects and Social Applications Set – Volume 4)

CORDELIER Benoit, GALIBERT Olivier
Digital Health Communications
(Technological Prospects and Social Applications Set – Volume 5)

NADOT Michel
Discipline of Nursing: Three-time Knowledge

2020

BARBET Jacques, FOUCQUIER Adrien, THOMAS Yves
Therapeutic Progress in Oncology: Towards a Revolution in Cancer Therapy?
(Health and Patients Set – Volume 2)

MORILLON Laurent, CLAVIER Viviane
Health Research Practices in a Digital Context
(Health Information Set – Volume 4)

PAILLIART Isabelle
New Territories in Health
(Health Information Set – Volume 3)

2019

CLAVIER Viviane, DE OLIVEIRA Jean-Philippe
Food and Health: Actor Strategies in Information and Communication
(Health Information Set – Volume 2)

PIZON Frank
Health Education and Prevention
(Health and Patients Set – Volume 1)

2018

HUARD Pierre
The Management of Chronic Diseases: Organizational Innovation and Efficiency

PAGANELLI Céline
Confidence and Legitimacy in Health Information and Communication
(Health Information Set – Volume 1)

2017

PICARD Robert
Co-design in Living Labs for Healthcare and Independent Living: Concepts, Methods and Tools

2015

BÉRANGER Jérôme
Medical Information Systems Ethics

Printed and bound by CPI Group (UK) Ltd, Croydon, CR0 4YY

16/09/2026

14963088-0003